ACCEPT | REFLECT | COMMIT

Accept
Reflect
Commit

YOUR
FIRST STEPS
TO
ADDICTION
RECOVERY

ADAMS RECOVERY CENTER

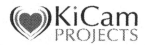

This book is not intended as a substitute for the medical
advice and care of physicians and mental health professionals.
The reader should regularly consult a physician and/or mental
health professional in all matters related to medical and
mental health care, including, but not limited to, the treatment
of addictions. The author and publisher hereby disclaim all
liability to any party for any causes of action arising from
reliance upon the advice presented in this book.

Cover and book design by Mark Sullivan

ISBN 978-0-9977222-9-1 (paperback)
ISBN 978-0-9985216-0-2 (e-book)

Printed in the United States of America

Published by KiCam Projects
www.KiCamProjects.com

CONTENTS

We are so excited you are holding this book right now. No, really. This is huge. Whether you are someone who has been struggling with addiction, you are the loved one of that person, or you just want to learn more about addiction and its treatment, this is a great step. We wrote this book for you, and you found it! That's awesome. So, let's introduce some things first.

WHY WE WROTE THIS BOOK

The fact is, addiction is widely misunderstood. At Adams Recovery Center (ARC), we speak with many confused family members and friends of our clients who cannot understand why their loved one cannot simply stop using. They don't understand why their loved one has stolen, lied, manipulated, and wrecked his or her life over a drug. It's confusing and hurtful. They want answers, and they want to understand.

This is common for the general public as well. Whenever a news article detailing an overdose, an accident caused by a drunk driver, or a crime committed by people addicted to substances is released, there is quick judgment. Look at how many communities petition against rehabilitation centers, detox clinics, or sober-living houses. They want people to get help, but not anywhere close to them. It's a classic "not in my backyard" mentality. And we get it. Addiction is scary. It's easy to see those news articles and make assumptions. The reality is, though, addiction is everywhere. It is in your backyard, your schools, your churches, and your shopping centers.

The other reality is that people who are addicted to substances also experience confusion. They wonder how their lives became so unmanageable and why they can't simply stop using. They might have been to multiple treatment centers and still find themselves returning to their substance of choice. They hear stories of hope in the recovery community and wonder why they can't seem to get it right. Unfortunately, sometimes they don't have the opportunity. The Centers for Disease Control and Prevention states that in the United States ninety-one people die every day from opioid overdose, and excessive alcohol use accounts for one out of ten deaths among adults.

It's becoming clearer and clearer that addiction is a life-or-death issue, and those seeking treatment and relief from these substances are fighting a very serious battle. We know, we know—we just got pretty intense! The reason for that, though, is because we are so passionate about helping people fight that battle. We have dedicated our lives to helping equip people with the tools necessary to live healthy, drug-free lives.

Within these pages, you will find information about the common thought processes and behaviors associated with addiction. If you're looking for highly technical and clinical information, this book might not be for you. We did not write this book for the clinician, but for the everyday person seeking to better understand addiction and its treatment processes. We wanted to make this information easily digestible and uncomplicated. We believe that, when it boils down to it, sobriety is simple. It's the problematic thoughts and behaviors that come with an addictive lifestyle that make it difficult.

We cover a wide variety of topics in this book, and they are all things we talk about daily with the clients at our treatment facilities. We've even thrown in some information about common thinking errors and thought processes that can make it difficult to move forward in sobriety, such as black-and-white thinking, instant gratification, and the victim mentality. We wanted to hit all the major areas we address with our clients and their families.

We don't believe this information is sacred or that you need to attend our facility to learn these "secrets." In fact, there aren't any secrets at all! There is no secret to sobriety. It's all about a true willingness to change and to put forth the consistent effort needed to make those changes last.

Our Program

ARC is an agency dedicated to change. We are a separate-gender drug and alcohol treatment program located in Clermont County, Ohio. We offer residential, intensive outpatient, and individual counseling services. Our program is a modified Therapeutic Community running the Hazelden clinical curriculum, and we use the latest evidence-based practices and incorporate cognitive behavioral therapy, rational-emotive behavior therapy, and behavior therapy to maximize client gains in the program. Our inpatient program is designed for an approximate 180-day stay. Our staff includes drug and alcohol counselors and mental health counselors.

ARC embraced the Therapeutic Community model due to its renowned success worldwide. The Therapeutic Community is a model recognized and endorsed by the United States federal government. Within the T.C., clients (called "sisters" or "brothers" and as a collective referred to as "the family") come out of their denial and into acceptance regarding their substance abuse. Clients expose their thinking errors and learn how to look at people, places, and things in a different fashion. The T.C. is a residential hierarchy in which every resident has a job (for example, cleaning the kitchen, taking out the trash, inspecting the dorms, etc.). Clients engage in five hours of group therapy per day, one hour of individual counseling per week, and case management as needed.

We do not believe that one size fits all when it comes to treatment, and we do not believe we can simply hand clients the answers. Instead, we help them find their own.

We do believe in the importance of sober support and family involvement, which is why we run a weekly family group and visit on Saturdays. Family members educating themselves on addiction and making their own changes are often an important component to our clients' treatment. That's why we promote this book for family members, too. Many of the concepts in this book are not addiction-specific, but human-specific. Unfortunately, as humans, we are not perfect. A lot of the information in this book can help each of us get that *little* bit closer, though.

When a client has made sufficient evident clinical and personal progress at ARC, the client graduates and is referred for aftercare. We make sure our graduates feel comfortable and confident in themselves and in their aftercare plans. We've had many clients go on to live successful lives free of substances, and we love hearing from these clients and celebrating the continued progress they've made.

Not every client who attends ARC graduates, though. No program can guarantee 100 percent success. Many programs exist, and many models exist, but in the end, it's up to the person going through the program to put in the work and benefit from what she or he learns.

Throughout this book, we will address the roadblocks many clients encounter and how to overcome them. We also will share client stories so you can see how these concepts look in real life. In order to protect the identities of these clients, names and some details have been changed. But that does not make their stories any less real or impactful. It's also important to remember that these are *their* stories, just as your story is *your* story. Comparing your journey to another's will not help you (more on that later). Use these tales as inspiration and guidance, not mandates.

OUR STAFF

The staff at ARC comprises individuals who are certified or licensed in various disciplines. All clinical staff hold, at the bare minimum, certification as a chemical dependency counselor in the state of Ohio (Chemical Dependency Counselor Assistant). Most staff are licensed as chemical dependency counselors (Licensed Chemical Dependency Counselor, Level 2 and Level 3), and others hold the Licensed Independent Chemical Dependency Counselor (LICDC). Multiple staff members hold the LICDC-CS, which is the clinical supervisory endorsement—the highest form of chemical dependency licensure in the state of Ohio.

We have a Licensed Professional Counselor (LPC) who is certified in the state of Ohio, and our medical coordinator is a Registered Nurse (RN) and holds a CDCA.

We come from various counseling backgrounds, from a variety of schools of thought. We draw from cognitive behavioral therapy; behavior therapy; rational-emotive behavior therapy; reality therapy; choice therapy; existential/gestalt therapy, etc. We bring a diverse therapeutic orientation to the table, which allows multiple techniques and interventions to be used.

If you tally the years of experience of the clinical professionals at Adams Recovery Center, you approach triple digits quickly! We never take a generic, cookie-cutter approach, and we believe this diversity allows us to help clients reach their goals without being placed in a box.

As for myself, my name is Kayla Scoumis, and I am the clinical coordinator of the men's facility. I am a Licensed Professional Counselor in the state of Ohio and I am working toward obtaining the status of a Licensed Professional Clinical Counselor. I am also a Licensed Independent Chemical Dependency Counselor and am working to obtain my supervisory status.

I earned my master's degree in Mental Health Counseling from the University of Cincinnati, which I pursued in order to do exactly what I am doing now: help people help themselves. I decided to pursue my practicum and internship at Adams Recovery Center and fell in love with both the agency and its clientele. Every day I was inspired by the clients and the hard work they put into their programs, and I became passionate about the program itself. I found myself aligned with the Cognitive Behavioral Therapy model and appreciated that the program was based in it, but I also loved the flexibility. I believe that individualizing treatment and meeting the client where he or she is is crucial, and I'm proud to be part of a staff and an agency that is so dedicated to its clients.

As I wrote this book, I took into account everything I have learned from my peers and supervisors over the past several years. Though I put the pen to paper, the ideas and concepts in this book come from all of us. Each chapter was approached in the following way: *How would I talk about this with my clients? What are some viewpoints of my coworkers on this topic? What is the theoretical or research basis on this topic?* Reading this book is truly like attending our program in written form.

My Adams Recovery Center colleagues and I truly hope you find this book helpful. Regardless of what led you to picking it up, we hope you put it down having learned some valuable lessons. Whether it's pursuing sobriety with confidence, supporting a person in your life who is seeking sobriety, or just learning how to be a better human, this book can provide you with some guidance. Remember, though, that only you can make the changes, and only you can put these ideas into practice. We believe in you, and we are so excited for your new life!

CHAPTER ONE

The Tipping Point

If you're reading this book, we assume you have a lot of questions and are looking for some answers. For many of you, the most important questions might be: Do I have a problem? Does my loved one have a problem? These are big questions, and we are going to try to make it very easy for you to answer them.

The question of whether substance use is a "problem" for someone is a common one. This is especially true when the person using insists he or she does not have a problem. You know, she can *totally* stop using whenever she wants. Or, he uses by choice, not by necessity. For some, this might be true. Many people can drink a beer and not pick up another, or try a drug and not touch it again for a while—or ever again! But we are guessing this is not the case in your situation, especially if some of the issues you're facing match up with ones we will discuss in this chapter.

First, let's just say up front what we won't be talking about. We will not be telling you *why* people abuse drugs or drink excessively. If you are searching for this answer, we regret to say it is not one you will find easily. Many people might offer ideas—genetics, peer pressure, low self-esteem, etc.—but while those things certainly can be *factors*, the reason someone uses will be entirely personal to that individual. Addiction is not the same for everyone, and it requires personal reflection and work for someone to figure out what drives his or her use. Worrying about the "why" can become a huge distraction for people in treatment. They become so focused on the problem that they are unable to find solutions.

This is especially common for people in early recovery. They believe that getting to the "root" of their addiction and figuring that out first will allow them to move forward. This isn't necessarily the case. In fact, it is more typical for clients to discover those answers along the way rather than at the start. That's why we've chosen to use this book to discuss many of the issues clients tend to experience throughout their recovery journey.

So now that we have that out of the way, let's get started.

WHAT IS ADDICTION?
Addiction, by definition, is being physically and mentally dependent on something. Very, very few people intentionally become addicted to substances. They begin using for whatever reason, and then their brain changes. The substance begins to affect parts of their brain that are necessary for everyday functioning, and the brain adjusts to the presence of the substance. The brain then demands that substance in order to feel "normal," and mental and physical

symptoms arise until the person reintroduces the substance to the body. This is why many people *want* to stop using but find it very difficult to do so.

For most, a life of active addiction shifts away from "I like this!" to "I need this in order to exist." Although that's not *entirely* true, that's how it feels. Not only does the person feel he needs the substance to function physically, but he has begun to rely on it as a way to cope with everyday life. What's more, while in active addiction, the individual develops certain behaviors and thought patterns that align with his addiction. These will look different for each person, but it's important to acknowledge their development. In treatment, we help clients challenge these beliefs and actions in order to re-adapt to more productive ways of thinking and living.

That is a quick and simple explanation of addiction. It's certainly not entirely comprehensive, but it is all you need to know right now to better understand yourself or support your loved one. Acknowledging the humanity present within addiction is absolutely necessary. Anyone can become addicted to substances and can go from use to abuse. Finding the line between the two is easier than you might think.

Is It Really a Problem?

You can determine whether substance use is a problem with one question:

Is your use, in any way, having a negative impact on any aspect of your life?

Yep, it's really that simple. If substance use is causing harm to any area of your life, it's something you need to look at. "Casual" use does not cause problems. It does not destroy relationships and careers. It does not come with multiple legal issues. There's little point to debating what "casual" use is. Just ask yourself that question: "Is substance use having any kind of negative impact on any aspect of my life?"

If you answered "yes" to this question, or if it applies to your loved one, we really hope you continue reading.

Let's review how professionals in the field view substance use. When assessing substance abuse and determining whether it qualifies as a disorder, we turn to the *Diagnostic and Statistical Manual of Mental Disorders (Fifth Edition),* more commonly known as the DSM 5. This book is essentially a manual of every mental illness and disorder, their symptoms, and other important information. The DSM 5 includes diagnostic information for all of the major categories of addictive substances and breaks down what could qualify the use as problematic.

In the DSM 5, substance abuse is assessed by the following factors:

1. The substance is either taken in larger amounts or for a longer period of time than initially planned.
2. The person has an inability to control or cut back use despite his or her efforts.
3. The person spends a significant amount of time trying

to obtain, use, and recover from the substance.

4. The person feels cravings for the substance.

5. The person is unable to follow through on responsibilities at home, work, or school due to his or her use.

6. The person continues to use despite experiencing problems with himself or herself and with relationships due to the use.

7. The person stops engaging in activities he or she used to enjoy due to the use.

8. The person consistently places himself or herself in risky situations in order to use.

9. The person keeps using despite physical and/or psychological problems caused or made worse by the use.

10. The person has developed a tolerance to the substance and needs to use more in order to feel the effects.

11. The person experiences withdrawal symptoms or uses in order to avoid withdrawal symptoms.

Here's the thing: The presence of only *two* symptoms can qualify someone for a diagnosis of substance-use disorder.

Keep in mind, though, professionals are looking for more than just a list of symptoms when rendering a diagnosis. That's why we want to make it clear that you should *not* diagnose yourself. However, if you can relate to any of the above symptoms, we encourage you to seek help. Even a "mild" use disorder is still something to address, because if ignored, it can progress into a more severe issue. How many people who struggle with alcohol addiction began with "just" using on the weekends? How many people who are now using heroin began by taking an extra pain pill after surgery? The thing with addiction is that it can progress quickly.

We understand that some of this information might sound scary, and it might even be confusing. Basically, just remember this: If your use hinders your life in any way, or if your loved one's use is hindering his or her life, don't be afraid to seek help. In the next chapter, we will explore different treatment options available so you can begin thinking about what might work for you or your loved one.

Before jumping to treatment, though, there are a couple of other issues to think about and understand.

INTERVENTIONS: FACT OR FICTION?

The concept of interventions has become popular over the years, thanks to TV shows and other media shining a light on them. They are usually presented as emotionally intense meetings, with the person being helped breaking down in tears and agreeing to go into treatment. This is a heavily edited and highly romanticized description of an intervention, but the positive is that it helped solidify the idea that family and friends can come together and encourage someone to better his or her life. Though each person's addiction is different, it is not solely an individual issue. It's more often a dynamic one that affects multiple people in a family or social circle.

Often people struggling with addiction might not

recognize the extent of their problem. Or they might not see how their addiction is affecting those around them. One common thinking error experienced by many in active addiction is the belief that their use hurts only themselves. Bringing people together to challenge those ideas and help a person see his or her value can help someone find the strength to seek treatment.

There is not much research on interventions because they are a difficult thing to study. Most of what we know about the effectiveness of interventions comes from case studies, real stories of people who utilized this tactic. Interventions can be effective if done right, but they are not guaranteed. We are talking about humans here, and they can be unpredictable, especially when substances are brought into the mix.

One thing we have found is that an intervention tends to be more effective if a professional is involved. That's because interventions can become emotional. Enlisting a professional to help guide the conversation can ensure that things remain on track and emotions do not run the show. Another thing to keep in mind is the importance of not yelling at or shaming the individual. Throwing blame or raising your voice might produce the opposite of the desired outcome, because the person might become defensive and not hear the message the group is trying to convey.

It's important to keep things specific. Make sure you are communicating your concerns in a way that provides examples. It's difficult for someone to deny something like "We have been late on every bill the past several months because the majority of our money is going to drugs" as opposed to "Your addiction is causing money issues."

Now, no matter how you present things, the person still might become defensive or angry. It's important to support your loved one in those emotions and let him or her know it's okay to discuss them with you. In short, keeping the conversation as focused, specific, and supportive as possible can make for a successful intervention.

ISSUES WITH INTERVENTIONS

If the intervention is not initially successful, it does not mean everything is ruined or you've failed. Sometimes it takes time for these things to sink in. We've had many clients say that they initially ignored their family and friends' concerns until the reality smacked them in the face somehow. With addiction (and with any hard thing, really), people truly have to want to deal with it. They have to want sobriety and have motivation within themselves to pursue it and embrace it. It might be easy for a person to agree to treatment when her loved ones are encouraging her, but once that addicted brain kicks in during treatment, she might abandon her promises.

One of the most important factors of a successful intervention is follow-through. This does not just mean for the subject of the intervention, but for the family members as well. For instance, if an ultimatum was given that the person either needs to enter treatment or he will be kicked out of the house, then there needs to be real consequence. Either the person goes to treatment, or he has to leave. Setting and maintaining clear boundaries is very important for all relationships and can be beneficial when trying to help those in active addiction. You might be scratching your head—how does kicking someone out of a house *help* him? Let us explain.

ENABLING: LOVING SOMEONE TO DEATH

Many loved ones of those struggling with addiction struggle with their own problematic behavior: enabling. Enabling means giving someone permission or ability to do something. When used in this context, it means allowing your person to continue doing what she has been doing without any real consequences. You are giving her permission and ability to continue with her addictive lifestyle by not setting boundaries that communicate it is not acceptable. You are making it easy for her to continue using because she is not having to perceive her use as an issue.

For instance, Mom, angry that her son is high, exclaims, "If you don't stop what you're doing, I'm kicking you out!" Mom, however, never actually kicks her son out. Son learns these are nothing but empty threats and ignores them, continuing to have a free and comfortable place to stay. Because he is not worried about shelter, he continues to spend his time and money on drugs. Now, if Mom actually followed through, Son would have some issues to resolve.

Where will he go? How will he pay for it? This is a major inconvenience!

That said, we are not implying that if Mom takes the hard line, Son will instantly embrace a life of sobriety. But here's the thing: Mom is no longer making it easy for him. She is no longer enabling his addiction by allowing him to engage in it around her. Mom communicated a boundary and followed through.

Here is where things can get messy: Son becomes very angry with Mom, and then Mom feels guilty. Mom, we totally hear you. We feel you. We promise we are not cold and heartless. Seeing your loved one struggle with addiction is a painful thing, and because you love that person, you want to help him. Enabling is not helping, though. It's slowly killing the person you love.

Enabling goes beyond allowing someone to live in your house. It also could mean giving him money despite knowing exactly where that money is going; allowing him to borrow your car despite the fact that he's wrecked several already while drunk; or calling in sick to work for him even though he's really just too high to go in.

Can you identify with any of those actions? Have you ever tried to set boundaries and then backpedaled out of fear that you might lose the person you love?

One of the hardest things to accept is that, if you continue to enable your person, you will eventually lose him or her anyway. Addiction can kill. It can, and it will, destroy everything in time. Being a pawn to your person's addiction will do nothing but destroy you as well. It is up to your person to recognize the need to embrace sobriety, and you cannot coddle someone into it. It might take him or her a long time to realize that, and that's the unfortunate truth of addiction. In the meantime, learn to take care of yourself. Seek help for the turmoil this situation has put you through. Connect with people who have been through similar situations so you can support one another. Find healing in knowing you are not directly providing your loved one a means to his or her possible end. These are all easier said than done, but it is important for you to recognize that you still matter.

Many of our clients cite their loved ones' setting boundaries as the reason they decided to seek help. For instance, one woman told us her mother refused to pick her up one night and she had to sleep on the streets. She said the experience was so traumatic that she realized she needed to get help. Boundary-setting does work, and it will be more helpful to your person than enabling is.

So Now What?

In this chapter, we've discussed what addiction is and what classifies use as a problem. We've reviewed interventions and provided some tough love on enabling. We recognize that we threw a lot of information at you in this chapter, and some of it might have been intense or upsetting. To be honest, though, you need to get used to that. This book is not going to sugarcoat things, because addiction doesn't do that. It's real, and it's raw. It takes away, and we are hoping to help you regain. So feel free to take your time with this book. Really soak it in. Revisit concepts that struck you or that didn't quite sit right. We cover a lot of ground in these pages, and we want you to get the most out of it.

If you're ready, though, keep going. We will review some treatment options with you and give you some ideas for how you or your loved one can begin pursuing a new life of sobriety.

• • • ALLIE'S STORY • • •

Allie entered treatment unsure if she "belonged" there. She was reluctant to open up to others because she did not feel she could connect with them. Allie was primarily in treatment for receiving her third DUI charge and was facing serious legal repercussions if she did not seek help. Allie struggled to identify her drinking as a problem because she was able to maintain a job and take care of her children during her use. Allie also described her use in the following way: "Only at night, after my kids go to bed. Then on weekends I like to have a little fun. It's what helps me unwind! I work hard, and I deserve it."

During a group process we have in our program, Allie began to see the reality of her situation. She recounted how her daughters would often be the ones getting her up in the morning due to her waking up hungover. She recalled how she would look forward to her nightly drinking and become irritated with her children when they didn't go to bed on her schedule. She acknowledged how she rarely spent time with her kids on the weekends because she was either out partying with friends or sleeping during the day. She admitted that she rarely put money into a savings account because all her extra funds went to buy alcohol.

Allie previously had believed her DUIs were just "bad luck," but she came to realize that they were the results of a larger problem. Once Allie recognized that her use was causing her problems, she was able to begin doing real work to develop new and more effective coping skills.

FOR REFLECTION

- Return to the chapter's central question: *Is substance use, in any way, having a negative impact on any aspect of your life?* How would you answer that for yourself?

_____

_____

_____

_____

- Reflect on what drew you to purchase this book. What questions are you hoping to answer? On what issues do you need guidance or resolution?

_____

_____

_____

_____

- Are you enabling your loved one's use? Is someone enabling your use? What boundaries or consequences might be needed as next steps?

  _____

  _____

  _____

  _____

CHAPTER TWO

Choosing the Right Treatment

The process of selecting a treatment option can be intimidating and even frustrating. There are so many choices—different types of treatment, various centers to call, dozens of factors to consider. The Internet is not always helpful, either. Websites that feature smiling people and promises of recovery don't necessarily comfort you. What will work best for you and your needs? You might not even know what to look for.

This process definitely can feel like a burden. Different treatment centers have different philosophies, different requirements, and different payment methods. Due to the current epidemic, most centers also have wait lists. All of this can feel discouraging to people seeking treatment, and the desire for sobriety might seem like a hopeless cause.

Despite the frustrations that can come with seeking treatment, it's still a worthwhile endeavor. In this chapter, we will go over several different types of treatment so you can get an idea of what might be a good option (or options) for you and start streamlining the process.

REALISTIC EXPECTATIONS

First, let's talk about the elephant in the room. When it comes to choosing a treatment center, you need to be realistic with your expectations. Movies and TV haven't done any favors to drug and alcohol treatment because they present it as a vacation with a little drama mixed in for fun. You can see it in your mind's eye, right? A luxe facility with a bunch of wacky oddballs who "find themselves" through solemn walks on the beach. Although the whole beach-and-luxury-treatment thing does exist, that does not mean it's the right facility for you, and those options are few and far between anyway.

Let's also take into account affordability. Insurance coverage might be a huge factor in what type of treatment you can seek, because self-pay can be very expensive. Making sure you choose a treatment option that is within your means can ensure that you will not have to leave prematurely, graduate treatment with a mountain of debt, or create a large financial burden on your family or friends. Now, if you do not have insurance, do not become discouraged! Some local social services agencies, such as Job and Family Services, can assist you with obtaining coverage.

Also, recognize that no treatment option is perfect. No facility, program, curriculum, staff, or treatment type is flawless, and there might be some things about it you don't like. If you stall on committing to a treatment type because you're focusing on small details that aren't ideal, you're only continuing to hurt yourself. Recognize and accept now that choosing the *best* treatment for you does not mean choosing the *perfect* treatment.

And last but not least, remember that no treatment type or program is a guaranteed "cure." Addiction is extremely complicated, and it requires a great deal of work to address. Some clients enter treatment expecting to be "fixed" and given all the answers to their problems. When that's not the case, they become angry and resentful, claiming the program isn't meeting their needs. In reality, they aren't putting in the work to find their own answers. Treatment provides you with the space to process and the tools to better your life. You're the one who must utilize the tools and put them into action. No one else can do that for you. A program is only as effective as you make it.

Now that we have all that out of the way, let's get to some treatment options.

DETOXIFICATION

This is the most basic type of treatment. Its focus is to assist the individual with detoxification from substances. Several substances can have terrible withdrawal symptoms, and this can make it difficult to embrace sobriety. Physical dependence upon a substance can prevent someone from stopping his or her use, even if he or she wants to quit. Many clients leave treatment within their first several days because the withdrawal symptoms feel impossible to endure. In fact, withdrawal from alcohol and benzodiazepine dependence can even be deadly, so medical detox is highly recommended for individuals who abuse those substances.

Detoxification programs medically assist clients with safely detoxing and keep them comfortable during the process. The benefit of detox programs is that they make the withdrawal period less terrible for people seeking sobriety. The downside to these programs is that they are often very short, usually from three to fourteen days. Typically this is not enough time for people to fully process and change the thoughts and behaviors that supported their use in the first place. However, detoxification programs are often a great first step—one that helps someone get over that first hump of sobriety in order to begin pursuing other goals or treatment options.

OUTPATIENT TREATMENT

With outpatient treatments, an individual visits a group and/or counselor weekly. In these sessions, clients can discuss and learn about ways to decrease their addictive behaviors and process issues related to their use. Some programs might require multiple sessions a week, whereas others are once weekly. Different programs have different philosophies. Psychoeducation—educating clients about issues related to addiction—might be the sole focus for some, whereas others might prioritize groups in which people discuss their weekly struggles. Others might combine these two or have different approaches. Seeing an individual counselor who specializes in addiction treatment is another form of outpatient service and can be helpful for people seeking one-on-one treatment rather than group support.

Outpatient treatment is ideal for someone who has stopped her use and has the proper support in place to be dedicated to treatment. We tend to recommend this type of treatment for people who have been sober from all substances for at least three months or who recently have graduated from a residential program and are seeking outside accountability. It will be difficult for someone to benefit from outpatient treatment if that person is actively using and/or does not have reliable means to attend her sessions. Also, if treatment is primarily focused on stopping use, the patient doesn't have much opportunity to process the thoughts and behaviors related to use, which greatly limits the effectiveness of the treatment in the long term.

RESIDENTIAL TREATMENT

Residential treatment is an option in which a person lives at a specialized facility for the duration of his or her treatment. Residential treatment centers can range from short-term to long-term stays and offer a variety of philosophies. Residential treatment is a great option for people who have difficulty maintaining sobriety on their own and need more structure. This level of care is also helpful for those whose home environments might not be suitable for supporting recovery. Residential treatment allows people to stay in a safe and stable place and provides them an opportunity to focus on themselves.

Treatment facilities vary in what types of day-to-day activities they provide and what treatments they offer. Because every residential program is so drastically different, here are some things to contemplate when looking for a residential program:

1. Structure: How much structure does the program provide? Is there a daily schedule that is enforced? How are clients held accountable for their actions, if at all?

2. Program type: What type of program does the facility follow? What counseling background(s) do they follow? Is it cognitive-behavioral? A therapeutic community? Twelve-step-based? A specific curriculum, such as Hazelden or Thinking for a Change?

3. Counseling: What type of counseling will be provided to you? Will you have an individual counselor? How often will you meet? Is group counseling utilized? What types of topics do they cover?

4. Interactions with others: How much interaction will you have with other clients? What will your responsibility be to them? Are you required to hold one another accountable, or is everyone working on a strictly individual program?

5. Facility: Does the facility appear well-maintained and safe? Is it kept clean? Who cleans it? Where does the food come from? How is laundry done? Where will you sleep?

6. Privileges: Are there any privileges of the program, such

as home passes or having the ability to work? What does communication with outside support look like? Are letters allowed? Phone calls?

These are some areas we believe are important to consider when thinking about entering residential treatment. Ideally, most of this information will be provided on a program's website, but don't be afraid to ask additional questions via phone, email, or an in-person visit. Call around and get more information. Schedule an assessment and see the place yourself. Again, no place will meet all your preferences, and you might even need to travel a bit to find one you feel good about.

There are some drawbacks to residential treatment. For one, living at the facility could be difficult for people who have young children or others for whom they are responsible. Another downside is the potential cost. Residential programs can be expensive if they are not covered by insurance. Check with your insurance provider to see what types of treatment your policy covers.

Medically Assisted Treatment

One option becoming more widely available for people struggling with addiction is medically assisted treatment (MAT). MAT utilizes medication to assist with withdrawal symptoms and/or cravings. MAT usually requires outpatient or residential programs so clients also can address any interpersonal issues related to their addictions.

Currently MAT is available primarily for those struggling with opioid and/or alcohol addiction. There are several types of medication available, and we will highlight three common ones here:

1. Buprenorphine is essentially a low-dose opioid that assists people with feeling less of an impact from withdrawal symptoms and cravings. It comes in pill and sublingual-film form. Taking buprenorphine also blocks the effect of any opioid, which can discourage people from using opiates. Though buprenorphine is an opioid itself, its effects are much weaker than prescription pills or heroin. There is also a low chance that those taking buprenorphine will become addicted to it, so it can be prescribed and taken by the individual at home or in a residential facility. There are risks to buprenorphine, though. Just because there is a low chance of becoming addicted does not mean it is impossible. Buprenorphine use also can come with some uncomfortable side effects and can produce withdrawal-like symptoms when use is ceased.

2. Methadone is similar to buprenorphine in the sense that it is an opioid and can be administered to assist people with withdrawal symptoms and cravings. It comes as a pill and an oral concentrate. Methadone is potent, which makes it an effective choice for those who experience severe withdrawal or who need pain management. Methadone does have a high potential to be abused, so

it is administered through clinics that clients visit daily. Unlike buprenorphine, methadone does not block the effects of opiates, thus increasing the ability to continue using while taking it. Methadone also can have uncomfortable side effects and intense withdrawal symptoms.

3. Naltrexone can be taken either as a pill or a monthly injection. Naltrexone completely blocks the effects of opiates, which might deter someone from using them. Naltrexone also cannot be abused because it does not produce its own euphoric effects. Naltrexone does not completely block the effects of alcohol use, but it does interrupt the pleasurable feelings that can come with drinking. Naltrexone also has few side effects.

People who enter treatment often question whether they should utilize medically assisted treatment. MAT is attractive for several reasons. First, withdrawal can be scary, so the idea of assistance through that process is highly appealing. People also take comfort in the fact that these medications can deter their cravings.

There are some drawbacks, though. People and their families often worry that using MAT is "replacing one drug for another." For some people, this is true in the sense that they become dependent on their MAT. Side effects are another concern with MAT. We encourage people interested in MAT to research all their options and to speak with a medical professional to determine if MAT is an appropriate choice.

SOBER SUPPORT GROUPS

Although they are not a form of formal treatment, support groups are very popular in the recovery community, and for good reason. They provide an outlet for people struggling with addiction to connect with peers and gain guidance in pursuing sobriety. People are attracted to sober support groups because of the sense of community they can foster and the ability to learn through others' experiences. There are many types of sober support groups out there, such as Alcoholics Anonymous, Narcotics Anonymous, Celebrate Recovery, SMART Recovery, Secular Sobriety, etc. Each type holds multiple meetings a day, multiple times a week, in multiple locations. One of the goals of these groups is to be easily accessible. Meetings normally cover a range of topics and issues so members can explore multiple areas of addiction and sobriety.

Each group has its own philosophies and approaches to sobriety. Most provide steps or guidelines for members to follow in order to work through their issues related to addiction. Many groups also host social functions so members can connect with one another and build healthy friendships. Sober support groups can be effective, but they do have their weaknesses. Because they are not clinically informed, sober support meetings might not have enough resources or support for people struggling with severe issues, especially if mental illness is involved. Another potential drawback is the one-size-fits-all approach some communities adopt, meaning a person's individual outlook or needs might be rejected. Also, as with outpatient treatment, if a person continues to struggle with active addiction, he might not receive the full benefit of meetings because his primary issue is stopping his use, which might require a higher level of care.

SOBER LIVING

Similar to support groups, sober-living facilities are not considered formal treatment, but they are worth mentioning. Sober-living communities are group homes for people in recovery; generally, residents must follow certain rules and contribute to the community by performing tasks or chores. People enter into sober living for multiple reasons and in various stages of recovery. Some might enter entirely new to sobriety, while some might have months or years under their belts. Most people choose to enter sober living because they are seeking structure and support from peers who are experiencing similar struggles and triumphs. Some sober-living facilities are very relaxed with few guidelines, while others might have many regulations in place. Some facilities even require residents to attend meetings or be enrolled in outpatient treatment. Sober living can be a great step for people who want to work and live a "normal life" yet still have reinforced structure.

Sober living does have limitations. The houses that have fewer rules and requirements might foster unhealthy or enabling environments in which people are continuing to use despite being in sober living. Some houses also might lack the funding necessary to maintain the facility and keep it safe. Also, sober-living houses might not be able to support clients who have more serious mental health or medical needs.

WHICH ONE IS BEST?

No treatment is considered "best." The best treatment is the one that resonates with you—the one you believe will work for you. Also, you don't have to pick just one. The majority of our clients utilize several—if not all—of the treatment options we have outlined in this chapter. Research does find that a combination of treatment types can be more effective for sustained sobriety. But remember, that does not mean that is what you have to do.

For more guidance, we recommend that you set up an appointment to have an assessment done at a social services agency. Some agencies even exist solely to assess and assist people with finding placement in treatment. In an assessment, you meet with a professional who asks you a series of questions related to your use. Ideally it will be conversational and allow you to fully express how your use has negatively affected your life. Once all the questions are answered, you will be recommended a level of treatment that can best meet your needs.

We hope that you found this chapter helpful and that you now have some idea of what direction you might pursue. Seeking treatment can be difficult, but we believe that, eventually, everyone can find an option that helps change his or her life.

• • • JOHN'S STORY • • •

John arrived for his assessment appearing irritated. When the assessment began, John insisted that he was not here for "rehab"; he believed outpatient treatment would be best for him. Throughout the assessment, John shared how his drinking had been highly detrimental to his life. He discussed how it affected his family life, his job, his friend-ships, his health, and his mental health. As he answered each question, John's mood quickly changed from irritated to depressed.

At the end of the assessment, the counselor reviewed John's assessment with him and pointed out some concerns. It appeared drinking had negatively affected every aspect of John's life, and John was unable to stop on his own. The most alarming factor was that John's drinking had sent him to the hospital for extended stays eight times in the past six months.

The counselor suggested that John enter residential treatment so he could more intensely work on his issues related to drinking and be in a safe place. John was disap-pointed, but he agreed to try it. Because John had been drinking heavily, he first attended a detox program so he could safely withdraw from alcohol in a controlled environment.

When his withdrawal period was over, John entered residential treatment. At first, he struggled to adapt to treatment, but he eventually began to make positive changes. As John neared the end of treatment, he feared going home due to his tendency to drink alone in his basement. John decided that he might benefit from sober living and decided to pursue that option. He researched sober-living facilities with his counselor and found one that appeared to be a good fit. John graduated from treatment and entered into sober living, where he still lives today.

For Reflection

- List five things here you want to learn about as you research treatment options:

_____

_____

_____

_____

_____

- Think about the types of treatment options mentioned in this chapter. What appeals to you about each? What do you *not* like about each?

_____

_____

_____

_____

_____

Detoxification:

_____

_____

_____

Outpatient treatment:

_____

_____

_____

Residential treatment:

_____

_____

_____

Medically assisted treatment:

_____

_____

_____

Support groups:

_____

_____

_____

Sober living:

_____

_____

_____

- What are the most important factors for you in selecting a treatment route?

  _____

  _____

  _____

  _____

  _____

CHAPTER THREE

Trusting the Process

A common phrase we use at ARC is "trust the process." That phrase can create either comfort or frustration, depending on how it's perceived. "Trust the process" will take on different meanings for different people, but it does have some core qualities.

What exactly *does* it mean to trust the process? Essentially, it is believing that life is happening as it is supposed to—which is both incredibly simple and incredibly complicated.

It's recognizing that, although we do not always have control nor the answers to everything, things will work out how they should if we continue to practice right living. It's acknowledging and accepting that life will take its course and we have control over only a small percentage of what goes on in the world.

That's a simple answer but not necessarily a simple concept, right? Are you really expected to just give up all control of your life and put it into the hands of some unknown source? Well, yes and no. Let's break this down.

First, think about a time in your life when you *really* wanted something to happen. It felt like life or death! You pulled all the strings, made important decisions, and tried to move all the pawns into place to bring that thing to you. But then…it didn't happen, or it didn't quite work out the way you'd wanted. Do you have that moment in mind? Okay, keep it there. We will return to it soon.

THE QUESTION OF CONTROL

Now, back to trusting the process and why it is so relevant to treatment and sobriety. At this point, you might have figured out a potential treatment option and are deciding if it's right for you. The thing with any treatment approach is that you are about to begin some sort of pre-established program. Whether it is entering residential treatment, attending a group several times a week, or working a twelve-step program, you are about to begin something that has a set path and structure. Though your own journey will have its unique qualities, you will be following the guidelines already determined by the treatment program you choose. Therefore, it is crucial that it is a program you truly believe can work for you.

Think about a twelve-step program, for example. Why are the steps so effective for so many people? One reason is that they truly believe in the steps—their sequence, the meaning behind them, the simplicity of progression, and so on. They trust that process and believe in its ability to help them. In contrast, if you feel the steps are baloney, will you really work them? Will you truly put your maximum effort into their requirements? It's very unlikely. Whatever your treatment option, it will be only as effective as your level of belief in its effectiveness. It will work only if you trust whatever process that program lays out for you.

We find that clients often struggle with trusting the process in residential treatment because it is a total, twenty-four/seven experience. After years, possibly decades, of living a certain way, clients enter into a realm where they are encouraged to live an entirely different life. New rules, new standards, and a list of behaviors that are considered acceptable and unacceptable can feel overwhelming. Telling someone who just entered treatment to "trust the process" is like telling a fish out of water to just breathe. It may feel difficult or even impossible. *How can I trust a bunch of strangers? Do these people really know what they're talking about? Why the heck can't I eat Pop-Tarts after 10:00 a.m.?* These are a few of the questions that might cross the mind of someone who just entered treatment, and they are entirely normal. If you are pursuing residential treatment, you probably will have these types of questions and myriad more, and what your brain probably will want you to do is begin trying to take control.

Many clients struggle with the issue of control, and it can create barriers in treatment. You might be thinking to yourself that control is not an issue for you. If anything, you feel completely and totally out of control due to a lifestyle of addiction. That's valid to an extent, but let's really look at it. Consider all the times you did everything in your power to obtain your substance of choice. You might have stolen, lied, manipulated, hustled, sold valuable items—fill in the blank. By doing these things repeatedly over time, you have developed an issue with control. You have created a lifestyle that you need to ensure is controlled to a point where you are able to continuously obtain your alcohol and/or drugs. You've developed skills that allow you to manipulate those around you and your environment to support your addiction. This is not meant to shame you; it's simply to acknowledge that control and an addictive lifestyle go hand in hand—and when you are used to being in control, it can be very hard to give that up. Then you enter treatment.

As mentioned, a program will work only if a person believes it will work and trusts the process. Many people enter a program initially believing it will work, but then the control monster rears its head. It rejects the changes because they are different from how it has been doing things for years. It balks at the thought of doing things that are uncomfortable. It desperately wants to return to that comfort zone where it pulled the strings. It tells clients that they know better; they've got this; they don't need to listen to these people—because who knows them better than they know themselves, right? And then the patients leave before any progress can occur. Unfortunately, these individuals often experience a relapse because no real change has been made and they continue to do things the way they want. The only process they trusted was their own.

Those who find success in treatment and achieve sobriety are those who are willing to relinquish control. These are the people who fully recognize that the way they have been living is no longer productive and does not make any sense for their future goals. They crave the input and guidance of others. They are willing to do things that are difficult and even scary. They take steps toward a new life rather than desperately trying to hold onto one that has done nothing but degrade them. They come in committed and ready to try something new. They are willing to trust the process. These individuals are not perfect, and they have plenty of moments of doubt and frustration, but at the end of the day, they believe the program they are working is what will work for them. It is what will help lead them to and support a life of sobriety.

What Trusting the Process Is Not

One common misconception we address is this: Trusting the process does not mean kicking back, relaxing, and just letting the process *happen*. Just because we are encouraging you to relinquish control does not mean we are saying give up complete and total control of yourself as a human. It's more about recognizing what you have control over, what you don't have control over, and putting it all together to create a healthy life.

Acceptance is the shining star of this concept. Let's use goal-setting as an example. Effective goal-setting requires an individual to think of a specific thing he or she would like to achieve and the steps necessary to achieve it. But one aspect many people forget about is acknowledging what barriers might get in the way and how they can possibly work around those barriers. Trusting the process is similar. You have the overall ideal in mind, but you recognize and accept that life might have other plans. Does that mean you just hopelessly sit around and see life as futile? No! You keep living and working and striving toward that ideal while remaining open to the other possibilities life might have in store. If a curveball comes your way, you adapt and continue moving forward. A new ideal comes to mind and you strive toward that. The cycle continues.

As stated earlier, trusting the process means believing things will work out. For things to work out, though, we need to do work ourselves. We rarely receive a paycheck for doing nothing. When we put the work in, life will reward us.

REFRAMING YOUR PERCEPTIONS

Often being in treatment will feel confusing, frustrating, and at times even infuriating. Things will not always go your way. You might be held accountable for an inappropriate behavior. You might strongly disagree with a statement made by a group facilitator. Your sponsor might encourage you to continue working a step when you want to move forward. Situations like these are when the control monster might try to return or you might doubt the program to which you've committed. When these moments happen, here's what we encourage: Take a step back, look at the whole picture, and consider some (or all) of these questions:

1. What role is control trying to play in this situation?
2. In what ways could this be a valuable experience?
3. How can I learn and grow from this experience?
4. How can I apply this to my life outside of treatment?
5. In the long run, will this matter?

By considering some of these questions, you are challenging your perceptions. You are allowing yourself to reframe the situation and acknowledge that there is more to difficult experiences than your own discomfort or negative emotions. You are allowing yourself to reconsider that process and remember the trust you've placed in it. By doing this, it is easier to continue moving forward through reflection and get back on track with your treatment goals.

PUTTING THINGS INTO PERSPECTIVE

Now, let's consider that situation you identified earlier in the chapter. You know, the thing you really, *really* wanted. Now that you've read through some of the concepts in this chapter, what are your thoughts? How can you answer the questions above regarding that situation? Hopefully you have some new perspectives. Maybe you're able to identify what you gained *instead* of that thing, such as a valuable life lesson or a more meaningful experience. Perhaps now you are able to see the bigger picture and identify some reasons why obtaining that thing wouldn't have been so great after all. Ideally you're able to see the process at work.

Trusting the process is far from easy. It means acknowledging that we are not all-powerful and things will not always be the way we want them.

If you do not trust the program you decide to commit to, building a solid foundation for sustained sobriety will be difficult. It will cause you to reject concepts that could be helpful for you, and you might try to control areas of your life in ways that are detrimental. But by trusting the process, you have faith that, through the difficulty and confusion, if you continue moving forward and doing your best, you will reap rewards greater than you can imagine.

In the following chapters, we will continue to reference the importance of trusting the process and how it can further relate to some of the concepts we discuss. So keep these ideas in mind going forward and, well, just trust the process, okay?

• • • JOSH'S STORY • • •

Josh had put in a significant amount of work in treatment, made many positive changes, and was able to identify and confront some core issues that greatly influenced his addictive lifestyle. But before he finished the program, he received a job offer that would require him to leave treatment before a plausible graduation date.

Josh experienced significant difficulty during this time and became obsessed with trying to figure out the "right" answer. The control monster even briefly came out, and Josh attempted to manipulate staff into letting him graduate early. Instead, we encouraged him to take a step back from the situation and consider his goals.

After a lot of processing, Josh decided to remain in treatment and graduate at the proper time. He remembered his original goal, which was to complete something he set out to do—a rare occurrence for him in active addiction. He also remembered the priority his family placed upon his graduation and how leaving early might negatively affect his relationships.

Josh did graduate and was able to stand with pride in front of his peers and family. He also eventually found a job he found fulfilling and better than the original offer. Though the situation he was in definitely proved to be a challenge, he allowed himself to look at the bigger picture and keep faith in the process that had been truly working for him, rather than giving it up for a new and shiny one. He also put faith in the process of life by trusting that by doing the right thing and staying in treatment, things eventually would work out—and they did!

For Reflection

- When you read about trusting the process, what emotions do you immediately feel?

  _____

  _____

  _____

  _____

- Think about control. How do you feel about relinquishing control in order to get healthy or help someone else get healthy? What do you associate with the idea of giving up control?

  _____

  _____

  _____

  _____

  _____

- Recall from early in this chapter the thing you really wanted but didn't get. What was the outcome of that situation? Is there any way you can think about that scenario in a more positive light?

  _____

  _____

  _____

  _____

  _____

CHAPTER FOUR

Playing the Victim Role

Life is terrible. I've lost everything. I have no one. I've done so many horrible things and burned so many bridges. Is it even worth it to pursue anything anymore? Will I ever amount to anything? I mean, why should I even try? Things will never be different. I will just keep falling into the same cycles and doing the same terrible things because I am the worst. Might as well just go use.

Does any of this sound familiar to you? Have you ever allowed yourself to dwell on everything negative in your life to the point where it became a reason to use? Welcome to something we call the victim role, a mentality that can greatly hinder any efforts toward sobriety.

To assume the victim role is to adopt a way of thinking that essentially makes you feel and act helpless. You use both past and present negative events as reasons to beat yourself up and view yourself as having no control. Rather than trust the process, you believe the process actively works against you. To play the victim means you believe you have no agency over your own life. You see the world as acting upon you rather than you being an active individual within it. This type of thinking is dangerous for everyone, but it is especially dangerous for those in active addiction. The victim role presents a prime rationale to use alcohol and/or drugs.

THE VICTIM ROLE AND ENABLING

The victim role allows those in active addiction to manipulate others. The "victims" communicate the beliefs in their head in a way that convinces their friends or loved ones that life truly is as bad as they say. This allows the "victims" to obtain money, a place to stay, companionship, more of their substance...the list goes on. In short, the "victim" manipulates others into enabling him or her.

Because the addict is now getting what he or she wants, the victim role feels productive and successful, but in fact it creates a complicated situation in which a person lives in misery while using that misery as a weapon. This is one reason why the victim role is often difficult to move beyond—it definitely can have its advantages.

The thing to remember, though, is that the victim mind-set tells you you're not worth anything better. It wrestles you into a submission that you accept and tolerate. That isn't living. You are worth more than that. And you are much more than just a victim.

Whenever we explain this type of thinking to clients, we often get a chorus of "That's not me! I don't think I'm a victim!" Sure, you might not adopt that as an identity, but that does not mean you aren't adopting it in your thinking. The victim mind-set is sneaky. Very few people want to be victims; they don't proudly proclaim, "I'm a victim!" But they interpret every negative thing—and even positive things sometimes—as a personal attack and validation that the world isn't fair to them. They keep tabs on all the unsavory things that cross their paths and use them as fuel for the fire.

THE VICTIM WITH LOW SELF-ESTEEM

The victim role manifests in different ways and wears different masks. We often see the victim mind-set in clients with low self-esteem. In short, their main belief system is: "Bad things will happen anyway, and I deserve it, so what's the point of trying?" It's very difficult for such a person to develop and pursue goals because he does not believe he can accomplish anything worthwhile. But low self-worth is only the surface-level issue. Though self-esteem is definitely something that needs to be addressed, the victim mind-set is present in the deeper beliefs this person holds. His view of life lacks agency. He does not believe his actions will make a difference because, either way, it will all go bad. He sees himself as a victim of life and, in turn, is comfortable with that position because he believes it is where he belongs.

Some clients come to treatment with very little or no real support system. They might be homeless, have no money, etc. Sometimes these clients view their situation as deserved because of their actions in active addiction. They feel hopeless because they don't have the resources and support of others. They become depressed because they don't believe they can emerge from their current situation. They can't see the opportunity to take back control and better their lives, which inevitably keeps them stuck.

THE 'GOOD PERSON' VICTIM

The victim mentality also can appear in those who see themselves as good people in a bad world. These individuals believe they are good people just trying to do the right thing, yet nothing seems to work out for them. No matter what good they try to accomplish, life has other things in mind—and it's not fair. These individuals might come across as thoughtful and hardworking. They do so much for others! But as soon as their own wants aren't met, they find themselves depressed and angry. They may think to themselves, "I give everyone what they want. Why can't I ever get what *I* want?" These individuals are the caretakers and over-the-radar types who put on a front that their actions are born of good intent, when in fact they are more motivated by potential gain. When that gain is not realized, they become bitter and resentful. Their primary belief is that the world is not fair and they deserve a fair world.

That said, these "good guy" victims aren't necessarily selfish. In fact, they tend to engage in codependent relationships that probably began at a young age. The only thing they know for sure is that to receive validation or feel loved, they must give in excess. These individuals also probably began their substance use in order to fit in and find acceptance.

Just as with clients with low self-esteem, these victims feel a lack of control. They perceive their actions as good, but the reality is that they are usually investing in the wrong stock. People-pleasers are an excellent example. They will say and do all the "right" things and go out of their way for others, but once something doesn't go their way, they become spiteful. For instance, a client might consistently participate in groups and praise staff, and then when she is denied a privilege, she will think, *I'm here doing everything right, and they don't even see it. How dare they? It's not fair. I never get what I want.* That's a perfect illustration of the victim mind-set: hopelessness and lack of control.

THE VICTIM WHO HAS EXPERIENCED TRAUMA

Other clients have adopted the victim mind-set because they indeed have been victims of situations such as childhood abuse, domestic violence, sexual assault, war, and other traumas. These individuals have been through tragedy and have not healed fully. They hold onto their trauma in a way that defines them and hinders their ability to move forward. Don't get us wrong—these situations have a major impact on a person, and we are not saying they need to "just move on." What we are acknowledging is that, when some people experience trauma, it creates a belief that all they will ever be is a victim of that situation. This then translates to assuming a victim mentality across most, if not all, areas of life.

People who have been through trauma often adopt the belief that they are "damaged" in some way. They did not experience a "normal" life, so they struggle to feel normal. They find it difficult to relate to others because the regular concerns and difficulties their friends and family members experience do not match their own. These perceptions build up a distrust of others and the world. It especially creates a strong distrust of the process. They say to themselves, "How can I possibly trust a process that made me go through *that*? How can I trust anything, or anyone, in this world when I have been hurt so badly?" Using substances allows these individuals to feel more comfortable in the world. It blocks the painful emotions and memories and allows them to wear a mask of normalcy.

It is important to note that some people who experience trauma might be diagnosed with Post-Traumatic Stress Disorder (PTSD) or might experience its symptoms. Symptoms of PTSD, as recognized by the DSM 5, include, but are not limited to:

- Persistent, intrusive memories of the event
- Night terrors related to the event
- Flashbacks in which the individual feels as if the event is happening again
- Consistently negative emotional states or inability to experience positive emotions
- Reckless or self-destructive behavior
- Distorted beliefs about the self being damaged, to blame, etc.

(Post-Traumatic Stress Disorder is a serious mental illness that often requires specified and intensive treatment. If you or someone you know is showing signs of PTSD, please seek out a mental health professional.)

In treatment, PTSD symptoms often surface as clients engage in self-destructive behavior to alleviate their emotional pain. These individuals have allowed what they have been through to hold power over them. Their victim mentality has them believing that life will never get better and they will never be able to move on.

BEATING THE MIND-SET

As you can see, there isn't just one type of victim mentality. By fleshing out the different variations, you might be able to see how some (or all) of your own thinking involves a victim mind-set in some way.

Or perhaps you are thinking to yourself, *Nope. Still can't relate. I am a champion of life.* The truth is, we all assume a victim mind-set in one way or another at different times in our lives. So take a step off the pedestal and get real. Once you see the victim role for what it is, it's easier to fight against it.

There is no one true way to "solve" a victim mentality. There are a few general approaches, though, that we believe are worth discussing.

The first way is through *reframing*—directly challenging perceptions and thought patterns. Through reframing, an individual is encouraged to take a viewpoint he has toward something and try on new perspectives. For instance, a client might complain about the type of food that is served in treatment. One way we can reframe this is by challenging him to think of other possible perspectives people might have toward the food. The client, if willing, will then list some possibilities: "Well, I guess some people may think that it's not so bad.... I know one guy was on the streets before coming here and scrounging for food, so he's probably happy with it.... When I was a kid, my parents weren't really around, so I guess it's nice to have consistent meals..." By acknowledging other viewpoints and briefly adopting them as their own, people are able to understand how limited their vision truly is.

As we grow up, we slowly but steadily develop a window through which we view the world. It's easy to believe that our window is the one true window through which everyone looks, forgetting that everyone else has his or her own window built over a lifetime. It's also easy to forget that we can, at any time, throw a rock through our window and shatter all the views that no longer serve us. Reframing is one way of throwing that rock. By intentionally glancing out other windows, we are more aware of the smudges and cracks in our own. We are better able to recognize how limited our view is and figure out ways to expand it. The victim mind-set presents us with a dingy and small pane, with bars blocking our view. By challenging it and reworking our perceptions, we can have floor-to-ceiling shimmering glass.

Another way the victim role can be challenged is an extension of reframing. You might have heard of it. It's called gratitude.

We often encourage clients to make daily gratitude lists to acknowledge the things in life they appreciate. Sometimes clients are convinced they will run out of things to write down within several days. They often surprise themselves, though, and fill up entire notebooks by the time they leave treatment. By actively practicing gratitude, people are able to challenge the victim mentality that tells them everything is terrible and they are terrible and their lives are terrible. Gratitude is acknowledging that things are exactly the opposite and that, despite life's struggles, there are many triumphs as well.

One other way we challenge the victim mind-set is by encouraging and developing a sense of empowerment. To become empowered means to increase your sense of confidence and strength in your abilities. It means believing that you *do* have control over your life in many ways and refusing to adopt a mentality that places you in a position of "lesser." Empowerment can also bring clarity to your identity. When you see yourself as an active agent in your life, you begin to recognize and nurture strengths and parts of yourself you might have neglected in the past. In treatment, many clients discover abilities, talents, and interests they pushed aside for years. They are no longer adopting an attitude that suppresses them. Empowerment directly counteracts the victim mentality. It instills a belief that essentially says: "I can handle challenges that come my way. I am a competent and active agent within my own life. I can stand with pride and confidence in myself."

• • • ANGIE'S STORY • • •

Angie entered treatment after the end of a twelve-year romantic relationship. Within those twelve years, Angie had been beaten and emotionally abused on an almost daily basis. She began to use methamphetamine with her boyfriend because "it just made it easier to exist." After the boyfriend ended the relationship to be with someone else, Angie began living in homeless shelters and had very little. She developed a victim mentality that closely resembled the first and third types of victim roles discussed in this chapter; she was a victim of long-term physical and emotional abuse and she felt worthless, hopeless, and incapable of change. She saw herself as damaged and unlovable, and she believed that, for various reasons, she deserved those years of abuse.

Over time, however, Angie began to change. Through the help of her counselor and the community, she began to see positive qualities within herself. She began to reframe her experience as one that made her strong and resilient, and she began to heal from her past through various activities that focused on empowerment. Angie also ended up helping others by giving presentations on how to identify and reject abuse in relationships. She graduated the program feeling confident in herself and in her sobriety, and she is still doing well today.

It's important to note that the changes Angie experienced were slow. Often we see these stories of success and fall back into the victim role: *Why can't I make changes the way that person did? Why can't I reframe my perspectives that easily?*

The truth is that, like most changes, it takes time, patience, and effort to truly abandon the victim mentality, but it is possible. Once you begin to see the victim role for what it is and how it manifests within you, you can begin challenging it and telling yourself that its messages no longer have a place within your life. By allowing yourself to see all that life can be, rather than focusing on what it isn't, you are able to move forward.

FOR REFLECTION

- How have you seen the victim role play out in your life or in the life of a loved one?

_____

_____

_____

_____

- What is a negative belief you're hanging onto? How might you reframe that belief to see it from someone else's perspective?

_____

_____

_____

_____

_____

- Focus for a moment on gratitude. No matter what is going on in your life right now, challenge yourself to list five things for which you're grateful:

  1. _____

  2. _____

  3. _____

  4. _____

  5. _____

Wearing a Mask

"Who are you?" This is one of the simplest and yet most difficult questions to answer.

Now, we should make it clear that we aren't just looking for your name. We are talking about that meaningful question of true self—who you are at your core. What makes you a unique individual?

Many people stumble over their answer, unsure of what to say. It's a huge question and one that can be answered numerous ways. You might be contemplating it yourself, wondering how you would respond. Some people spend their entire lives searching for the answer. In a way, that's basically life, right? Stumbling around, trying to figure out your purpose and meaning...trying on different roles and hobbies and seeing what fits.

Something can happen in that process, though, that can be harmful, and it's pretty much guaranteed to occur while in active addiction. What we are talking about in this chapter is wearing a mask (or multiple masks) and why it is so necessary to unmask yourself.

Active addiction slowly but surely destroys a person's true self, leaving it crumpled and neglected. Years of thought patterns and behaviors that cater to obtaining and using a substance create an identity that is inauthentic. For instance, we have many clients who talk about morphing from a "good kid" growing up in middle-class suburbia to a "street thug" living in trap houses. Once they stop using, it might begin to feel weird using certain slang and dressing in a certain way. Without a substance masking the true self—those thoughts, feelings, and desires that have been buried for so long—a person often has no idea who he or she really is anymore. Clients often experience confusion and frustration over these identify conflicts, so a main goal in treatment is helping people meet themselves again and embrace the true person they've been hiding away.

MASKS VERSUS ROLES

Now, there is a significant difference between wearing a mask and catering to different life roles. As humans, we all have various roles. Some are naturally given to us, such as being a child or a sibling. Other roles are ones we willingly adopt, such as being a friend or choosing a career. These roles all have different needs and require different responsibilities.

We also adjust ourselves based on the expectations of these roles. For instance, the way you talk around your grandparents and the way you talk around your friends might be extremely different. With your grandparents, you probably clean up your language and filter some of the topics you discuss.

And sometimes roles conflict, such as when a work event

(role: employee) is at the same time as your daughter's recital (role: parent). Figuring out a balance of these roles and remaining true to your values and priorities is a natural and normal struggle of life. This is *not* what we are referring to when we talk about wearing masks.

The main difference between mask-wearing and role-catering is genuineness. Despite meeting the different expectations of each role in your life, you still remain true to yourself. You are the same person overall. It is one thing to filter your language and the topics you discuss around your boss. That's respectful and will help keep you from getting fired. It's a completely different thing to lie to your boss and say you can take on a project that requires a skill set you don't have. That's the kind of conversation you walk away from and wonder, "Why the heck did I say that? I'm in trouble…" That's wearing a mask. You wore the mask of a willing employee who can handle a big project because it would look good, and you're too proud to admit you can't do it. In the end, this might end up getting you fired when you drop the ball. Masks have a way of catching up to us because they don't have true substance behind them.

Masks and Manipulation

It would be impossible to identify every possible mask a person can wear, because masks are so individualized and have different motives behind them. One common thread, though, is that they are based on lies and manipulation. Think about it—why do we ever wear a mask? What advantage do we have to hide ourselves behind a façade? Why would we lie to our boss about our abilities, or to our partner about our whereabouts? When it comes down to it, we wear masks in order to manipulate. We want to control how others perceive us. We want to be seen in a certain way because it is advantageous for a particular goal. When we choose to wear a mask, we don't trust that our true identity will serve us in the way we want. Instead, we decide to adopt a different identity because it could get us something.

You might be able to see already how and why masks are so prevalent in active addiction. Let's use one example to illustrate how masks can be used to manipulate. One primary reason addicts wear a mask is to hide their use. It's rare that someone struggling with an addiction will want to willingly admit to his use, especially to those who would disapprove. It's common for us to hear family members talk about how they had no clue their loved one was using until it became obvious in some dramatic way. This is because that person wore a mask of living a "normal" life. For a certain period of time, he was able to keep his use a secret and adopt an identity that supported what he wanted people to think.

In other cases, people in addiction use masks to hide the severity of their use. How many times have you said, "I mean, I *only* use on weekends. It's not *that* bad," to others or possibly even to yourself? That's a mask. Do you see the lack of genuineness in these masks and how they hide the true reality of the individual? If this continues and the lies pile up, it's difficult to even distinguish reality from falsehood anymore.

Most individuals who enter treatment experience some sort of identity crisis. They've spent so much time catering to a certain identity that they can no longer separate themselves from the person (or people) they have pretended to be over the years. One way we encourage clients to begin removing their masks is to identify what their masks are and what they represent. There are so many different masks and identities a person can adopt. Treatment is an excellent time to begin getting to know your masks. What are they? What do they mean? How have they served you? What are you trying to hide by wearing a particular mask?

What Does Your Mask Do for You?

Let's look at this issue through the eyes of some of pop culture's most popular mask-wearers. Why do superheroes wear masks? Why is it so necessary for Superman to pretend he is just an average guy named Clark Kent? Or for Batman to don the suit and mask when he goes out at night to fight crime? The suit and the mask—symbols of an alter ego—are basically requirements in these universes. So why are they so bad in the real world? If Iron Man can wear a mask and be awesome, why can't everyone wear a mask and be awesome? These characters take on alternative identities because it provides them with the ability to achieve what they want to achieve. They wear masks to work toward the greater good and keep themselves safe. They know that if their true identity is revealed, it will be dangerous for various reasons. Each character's origin story reveals the weaknesses he possesses and the reasons he needs to hide his true self.

Let's really look at this, though. We idealize these super-heroes and the masks they wear, but that does not mean it makes sense for us. Superheroes wear masks because it allows them to save the world. It's a noble act, and even humble in a way. For us, though, it is the exact opposite. We are average people, and our masks serve no one but ourselves. We don't wear masks to save the world; we do it to save our own egos.

When we wear masks, we do so because we don't want to reveal our true selves, our vulnerabilities, and our insecurities. If anything, we wear masks because they help us feel like superheroes in our own lives, and we do not trust our true selves to get the job done.

This is a false belief, though. Wearing a mask actually hinders your ability to move forward. By throwing away your mask, you're allowing yourself to trust the process. You learn to trust that your true identity is the one that will lead you to the life you want, while a false one will only hold you back.

In our program, we have all clients write and share their autobiographies. This is a common practice in treatment centers, because it allows clients to see the impact of addiction on their lives. It is also a way for clients to explore their own origin stories. By writing out their lives and acknowledging the significant events that have shaped them, they are able to identify their own patterns, weaknesses, and strengths. They are able to see where their masks began to develop and how those masks have served them. It's one of those difficult yet necessary aspects of treatment that enables people to begin the journey of self-exploration. Many clients have been able to see what areas of their lives have caused them distress and how they have been hiding behind their masks for many years.

IT's TIME TO REVEAL THE TRUTH

Challenging and removing masks is something that takes work and effort. Yes, the autobiography exercise helps, but it's not as though someone can write his auto and totally understand himself. It's a lifelong process. It's also difficult to remove a mask that has been worn for so long.

Masking emotions is particularly hard to change. Many clients—really, humans in general—strive to keep their true feelings hidden. Typically a select few emotions are considered "acceptable" (happiness, for example, and sometimes anger), and anything outside of those emotions is shunned and bottled up.

This is especially difficult for those recovering from active addiction because substances have not only masked their emotions but also numbed them. When people first become sober, a flood of emotions usually overwhelms them. They often wonder if they are "going crazy." The mask begins to crack, which creates even more stress because they feel a need to keep it together. We often challenge clients on this, questioning why they choose to bottle the emotions that are begging to come out. The answer is usually centered around not wanting to look weak and/or not wanting to think about or accept the reasons for the emotions. Again, masks at work. Those masks are no longer serving the person, though. When we spend so much effort catering to something that no longer serves us, it becomes a burden. It's like a relationship that's run its course. At what point do you just admit it's time to break up? Here we're telling you: It's time to break up with your mask.

Embracing yourself for who you truly are is liberating. Yes, superheroes wear masks, but that's fiction, and you've been living in a fictitious world for far too long. It's time to enter into reality and see the world in its entirety rather than through two tiny holes.

• • • BRIAN'S STORY • • •

Brian came into treatment after several years of heroin addiction. He progressed well through the program but had difficulty letting go of one of his masks. This mask was one that made Brian appear helpful and caring. Brian was always there for other clients who were struggling and often had a joke to cheer them up. Brian was very giving and often stated that he found purpose in helping others. He graduated from the program successfully, but we unfortunately saw him again several months later.

This second time through the program was more

difficult. Brian had difficulty understanding why he relapsed. He came up with various theories but then would become frustrated because it didn't feel like "the answer." Through a lot of work in group therapy and with his counselor, Brian came to a realization. He started to see how wearing the mask of someone who is helpful and caring was not completely genuine. Yes, Brian was caring and helpful, but it was more out of a desire to please others than to actually help them.

Brian would often neglect his own needs or goals in order to make others happy. Sometimes Brian wanted to ignore others' wants. When he would have these thoughts, though, he would feel guilty, put his mask on, and act accordingly. This struggle between his true needs and his caring, helpful mask caused Brian to become confused and lost. He would use in order to cope with these feelings and punish himself for his "selfishness."

Brian began to realize that he was not selfish—that thinking of his own needs was necessary for good mental health. Through this understanding and growth, Brian was able to embrace his own wants and desires rather than always cater to those of others. He began to get to know himself and identify goals he previously had left untouched. This was especially impactful when it came to Brian's relationship with his parents, who had specific career plans in mind for Brian. He developed the courage to tell his parents that their goals were not his goals, and despite their displeasure, he stood his ground. Brian successfully graduated the program again, this time feeling more assured and confident in himself.

FOR REFLECTION

- Think about your masks. Do you see a hero, just trying to do the best you can? A villain, doing nothing but causing chaos for those around you? Maybe a victim who needs saving? Make a note of some, if not all, of the masks you wear.

_____

_____

_____

_____

- What do those masks do for you? For example, do they help you hide emotions or meet the expectations of others?

_____

_____

_____

_____

- Unmask yourself for a moment. What are some of the great qualities about yourself that you wish people could see? What parts of yourself do you most want to take out of hiding?

_____

_____

_____

_____

CHAPTER SIX

People-Pleasing

Very few people want to be seen as selfish. Helpfulness, politeness, and kindness are qualities people often strive to possess. People go out of their way to hold doors open for strangers, help clean up a mess, and even pick up a shift for a sick co-worker. These are all examples of actions that are viewed with reverence and respect. It's great to help others and consider their needs! When does that become a problem, though?

You might be scratching your head. Problem? How can being *helpful* be a *problem*? We call it people-pleasing, and we see it as a behavior that is harmful not only in action but also in its underlying belief and motive. People-pleasing comes in many forms, all of which have one thing in common: They are not actually beneficial for anyone, despite how it might seem on the surface.

People-pleasing is a challenging concept, because it's easy to dismiss certain actions as simply considerate behavior. We hope this chapter will help you see just how harmful people-pleasing can be and how it can hinder efforts toward sobriety.

It's Not All Good or Bad

This is a good time to introduce a concept we often discuss with clients. Black-and-white thinking is a common thinking error with which many clients (and people in general) struggle. It's a belief that something or someone is either one way or another, and there is no in-between. These types of thoughts usually incorporate words such as "always" or "never." For instance, maybe you've found yourself thinking something along the lines of *I'm such a failure. I'll never get it together.* By telling yourself this, you place yourself into an unfair and unreasonable box and destroy any motivation to "get it together"—whatever *that* means.

Black-and-white thinking also manifests in perceptions about the world, and it hinders people from being able to see and accept alternate views. In a way, it's almost an "us against them" mentality, a type of thinking that can be very dangerous. For example, it is often difficult for people in the recovery community to accept ways of maintaining sobriety different from their own. In treatment, we see clients who have different ideas about what their lives will look like post-treatment. Rather than use these differences to learn and grow, clients sometimes use them to create distance, to judge, and even to ridicule. One thing we encourage clients to do is embrace the "gray" between differing views. By doing this, they are able to build respect and create bridges between each other.

Clients usually enter treatment with some pretty solid opinions on how the world works and their place in it. More often than not, these beliefs are inaccurate and harmful. One of the best things a person can do is challenge the beliefs that hinder him and keep him stuck. Remember the window analogy from chapter four? That applies here as well, even though it can be difficult to change your world-view—especially when it comes to something like people-pleasing. It's hard to challenge a quality that you might perceive as positive. For many people struggling with addiction, their people-pleasing tendencies help them feel good about themselves. So, let's acknowledge something: Doing things for others can be good, *and* it can be bad. There is a lot of gray area here—it's not all one way or the other.

PEOPLE-PLEASING OR MANIPULATION?

People-pleasing can be detrimental, depending on the motivations behind it. We have many clients who are adamant that they help others because it is simply the right thing to do. But we challenge this and encourage clients to dig more deeply. Frequently they discover that their people-pleasing isn't about helping others—it's about benefitting themselves. It goes back to that common phrase, "I scratch your back; you scratch mine." By being overly helpful and kind, the person hopes that other people will feel more inclined to help her when she needs it. Such help can range from something as simple as sharing food to something more involved, such as providing money or shelter.

But what's the big deal? Isn't that just how the world works? Well, sure—sort of. For instance, when we hire someone to perform a task, we hand over money in exchange for that service. That's a mutually understood and beneficial situation. But we aren't talking about commercial exchange of goods. We are talking about regular people and manipulation. When a person is looking to manipulate another person, he is unlikely to directly communicate his intentions. What would he even say? "I'm doing this thing for you because I plan to use this against you later to get what I want"? No way! It's going to be discreet, and it's going to be sneaky. It's going to come back later, seemingly out of nowhere and will look more like this: "Wow. I helped you out three months ago and really put myself on the line, and you can't even do this for me? I can't believe you would do that. Shows what kind of person you are....Oh, you'll do it now? Great!"

Have you ever heard or said something similar? That's manipulative people-pleasing at work. When manipulation comes into play, it negates any good from doing a favor or being helpful. Truly good deeds are devoid of any intention to gain from them. So think about your intentions. When you do something for someone, is there a hope that he might do something for you in return? Even if it's subtle, it's important to acknowledge. By acknowledging the intentions, you are able to more clearly see how people-pleasing can be detrimental.

People-Pleasing and Street-Like Behaviors
People-pleasing is a common behavior on the streets and in jails. In those environments, money is either tight or

nonexistent, so people rely on the exchange of other goods or favors. For example, one issue we see in treatment is clients allowing their dealer to stay with them in exchange for drugs. It might start off with only the dealer staying there, but then he or she might move in a significant other, and then a friend, and then other people who buy from the dealer. Suddenly the client is essentially running a trap house. When he or she tries to address the issue, the dealer comes back with the fact that he has been supplying the client with free drugs. The client is stuck. That is how manipulative people-pleasing works.

The way we see this most commonly in treatment is with accountability. Clients will agree to not hold each other accountable for certain things in order to get away with breaking rules. For instance, one client will turn a blind eye to another not doing his chore in exchange for the other client ignoring him eating food in the dorm. They both do this thinking they are just doing a favor for a friend and helping each other get by—brotherhood and so forth. You might be thinking, *Wow, how does this even compare to the trap house thing?* At its core, it is still the same behavior and thinking pattern from the street. It's people engaging in an exchange based on dishonesty and potential harm. Though allowing someone to break a small rule in treatment might seem minimal, such things build up. When you get comfortable allowing small things to slip by, the larger things eventually become easier to ignore as well. Are you beginning to see how there is a lot of "gray" when it comes to people-pleasing?

"Snitches Get Stitches"

Another way people-pleasing can be present in street-like behaviors is the snitch mentality. The word *snitch* is one that traces back to our playground days. We learn at a young age that you don't tattle, because that makes you a snitch. It causes you to be an outcast. "Snitches get stiches." Most people eventually grow out of this mentality, recognizing it as childish and unsafe. There are simply some things you need to report. This might cause some people to be angry with you, but it's a risk you are willing to take.

Many people, though, hold onto this idea throughout their lives. It is especially present in jails and with people engaging in active addiction. Think about it: When people are engaging in illegal activity that is mutually beneficial, of course it is seen as unacceptable to "snitch" to the police or other authorities. There is a shared understanding that what they are doing is inherently wrong, but they have minimized, justified, and rationalized around it to feel more comfortable being in its midst. Many people will even go as far as being wrongly accused and accepting charges in order to honor the "snitch code." This is the ultimate form of people-pleasing, and it's highly enabling. This is also a great example of black-and-white thinking. Many clients struggle with letting go of the snitch mentality and have difficulty seeing the value in accountability. They have a black-and-white view that tells them they need to mind their own business or else they are in danger.

Now, we must acknowledge that snitches literally do get stitches in many situations on the streets and in jail. Addiction makes it easy to accept and tolerate such conditions. But when you're sober, or getting sober, there is no longer a need to accept this way of life. You no longer have to surround yourself with people who would physically harm you for holding them accountable. You no longer need to fear incarceration. Living a life of sobriety means being able to abandon these environments for good. When you change your environment, you also need to change your thinking and your behaviors.

TAKING OWNERSHIP OF YOUR ENVIRONMENT

When a person refuses to hold the people around her accountable out of fear of hurting someone's feelings or being labeled a snitch, she is choosing to prioritize people-pleasing over her own safety and sobriety. While in treatment, clients are encouraged to find strength in themselves to take initiative within their environments. Because our program is heavily community-based, we stress that it is primarily up to the clients to foster an environment that is therapeutic, trusting, and safe. We provide them with the tools to do this and help them put those tools into action. That is hindered when multiple clients engage in people-pleasing behaviors. They turn blind eyes to one another's behavior, join one another in teasing others or gossiping, and do not challenge one another to do the right thing. How much change can really happen if treatment is basically the streets without substances? When people take initiative and no longer tolerate harmful behaviors and thinking patterns in their surroundings, they slowly but surely build an environment that fosters growth and support.

That means doing things that might not make others happy. It might mean calling someone out for being manipulative, not allowing someone to slack on a responsibility, or encouraging someone to join you at a meeting when he doesn't want to go.

It will mean no longer prioritizing the happiness of others over your own needs and goals. In fact, sometimes it might even mean telling someone "no." It might mean not assisting someone because it conflicts with a task you need to do. This reality is a hard one for people to accept. In a way, it feels selfish, doesn't it? We receive different messages about self-care. One minute we hear, "Do what you need to do for you!" and the next we're told, "You need to consider others or else you're a jerk." It's confusing, and this is where that black-and-white thinking can come in. Let's look at this in more depth.

Helpful to a Fault

The recovery community values reaching out and helping others who are struggling. For those embracing a life of sobriety, this is appealing because they recall how others helped them in their times of need. They go out of their way to do things for others, such as sending daily encouraging text messages, providing rides to meetings, or buying someone coffee or a meal. Because they've made significant changes, they are no longer doing these things in order to manipulate. They genuinely want to help.

This is often a valuable, positive experience that allows people to get in touch with their sense of gratitude. It's great to help people, right? We've all struggled at some point, so we can see the benefit of getting and giving a hand up. The key is to keep things in balance.

When a person consistently places the needs of others above her own, it can take a toll. She might begin to neglect responsibilities, spend money she needs to save, or compromise her own emotional needs in order to help others. This is another form of people-pleasing, and we see it in treatment, too. Some individuals consistently set aside their own work in order to listen to someone's else's struggles or assist with a project. Usually this person realizes that she is not progressing because she is working everyone else's program but her own. She feels confused, though, because it seemed like she was doing the right thing. Here's the trick: While she was doing a *good* thing, was she really doing the *right* thing? That's the gray area, and there is no definitive answer. One thing we do know, though, is that a person has to take care of herself in order to take care of others. When a person doesn't take any time to recharge, how can she provide energy for those in need?

BE SELFISH

You have permission: Be selfish sometimes. Shape your environment into one that will support you and your sobriety. Set boundaries, even if they frustrate or anger others. Become comfortable with the word "no." Examine your patterns and behaviors and figure out when you tend to people-please. Is it to manipulate? To gain acceptance? To feel good about yourself? A mixture? Examining the motivations behind your people-pleasing behavior could assist you in kicking it to the curb. Remember: No amount of people-pleasing will keep you sober.

• • • BRENDA'S STORY • • •

Brenda entered treatment at the age of fifty-two after years of alcohol addiction. She entered into a community composed mostly of women ranging from ages nineteen to thirty-two, so Brenda quickly adopted a "motherly" role in the community. Her relationship with her own children was rocky due to her addiction, and providing that guidance and nurturing to the younger clients provided Brenda with a sense of purpose.

But Brenda's role became harmful not only for herself but also for the other clients. Brenda was reluctant to hold the other women accountable because she feared being rejected. She often excused their actions and cosigned harmful mentalities because she believed she was being supportive. Brenda also experienced anguish whenever a client would leave treatment prematurely. She would question what more she could have done, and her validation often relied on the success of others.

When her counselor would suggest that Brenda focus on her own issues and treatment, Brenda would reject this idea, stating, "Listen, these girls need me. If only you could hear how much I help them."

One day a client to whom Brenda was particularly close decided to leave treatment. Hours later Brenda decided to leave treatment as well, believing she and the other client could help each other in sobriety. Unfortunately, several weeks later Brenda called to say she had relapsed and wanted to re-enter treatment. She never made it to her assessment, and we are unaware of her current situation. We hope she eventually realized how her people-pleasing was harmful to her and is living a sober life.

FOR REFLECTION

- Have you engaged in people-pleasing behaviors before? What were some of your genuine motivations?

_____

_____

_____

_____

_____

- Recall a time when you were manipulated by a people-pleaser. What did the manipulator hope to gain from you? How did you feel in that situation?

_____

_____

_____

_____

- Write down an example of black-and-white thinking in your life. Now, if you change your perspective, what are some shades of gray you might be able to see?

_____

_____

_____

_____

- How do you feel about prioritizing your own needs? What do you think will happen if you start saying "no" to certain requests from other people? (Be on the lookout here for more black-and-white thinking.)

_____

_____

_____

_____

CHAPTER SEVEN

Avoiding Dangerous Comparisons

As humans, we are social creatures. We interact constantly with the world and the people in it. In doing so, we are consistently evaluating ourselves in relation to others, and that's okay for the most part. In fact, we've been doing it since we were kids. Think back to your childhood. If your sibling got a cookie, didn't you think you deserved one too? If your friend had a new bike, didn't you want one as well? Even when we are young, comparisons affect our emotional state. The thing is, comparisons among children tend to be simpler.

Then adolescence hits, and things get complicated. Preteens and teenagers, as they strive to find their identity in the world, measure themselves not only based on material items but also based on the qualities they possess and the acceptance they feel from others. They eventually find their group and want to act, dress, and think in ways that go along with that group. They compare themselves to one another for guidance. This is normal and natural. But this is also where the bigger issue begins. Often, people will use comparisons to set standards for themselves that are not realistic or achievable. They might even begin to alter their values to coincide with what they believe is more socially acceptable.

Adolescence is when we began to shape our view of the world, and we are still constantly shaping it as adults. What if we've created an unfair reality, though? One in which we place ourselves into a category of "less than" in relation to those around us? This is the world many live in, and it's one with which people in active addiction are very familiar. In this chapter, we are going to talk about dangerous comparisons and what they could mean for your sobriety.

Comparisons in Sobriety

When someone begins to pursue a sober life, he begins to re-explore his identity. It's similar to the questions asked in adolescence: Who am I? What do I like? Who will I become? Addiction takes away one's sense of self, and part of sobriety is figuring out who you are without your substance. Another way new sobriety is similar to adolescence is in the constant tendency to compare. Because you are trying to figure yourself out again, you're looking to others for guidance. That process can be dangerous if it's not kept in check.

One issue we see often with clients is comparison of progression. Clients will compare their different rates of progress in the program and use this as a way to boost or deflate their self-esteem. This type of thinking is very black and white and can prevent clients from focusing on relevant issues. Instead they're focusing on how they compare to others. We stress that everyone moves at his own pace and travels his own path, but this can be a hard concept to accept.

"IT'S NOT FAIR!"

Focusing on what is or is not "fair" is a common roadblock in treatment. There are milestones in the program that all clients accomplish, but they all experience them at different times based on individual progress. We often hear statements like, "Hey! He's only been here for thirty-five days and just read his autobiography, but I've been here for fifty and still haven't read mine!" Never mind that this client has written only two pages of his autobiography and has been disengaged from treatment despite staff support and encouragement. He wants to focus on the fact that "He got his before I got mine!" This is an example of how comparison allows someone to ignore the reality of a situation and instead take a victim stance. As we discussed in chapter four, dedicating emotional energy to this issue is a waste. This also relates to that childlike method of comparison—wanting something simply because you don't have it.

"I'M NEVER GOING TO GET IT RIGHT."

Clients also can draw dangerous conclusions when they compare themselves to other clients with similar issues. For example, two female clients were both struggling with a traumatic experience: Each woman had lost a child to illness. One client, through working with her counselor and completing assignments, had reached a point of acceptance over the event and had moved on to other issues. The other client, however, still felt wracked with pain and guilt. As she saw the other client move forward, she began to feel even more guilty and "broken." She wondered if she would ever be able to progress, and she questioned her program.

We helped her to realize that the other client's progress was completely irrelevant to her own. We also helped her reframe her expectations for what progress looks like regarding this issue. This is something anyone seeking sobriety should keep in mind: Having a particular expectation for how sobriety will look, or how you will feel while confronting an issue, might be more harmful than helpful, because your expectation is probably based on a comparison. In this case, one client believed that her progress, her acceptance, would look like the other client's. Her belief was inaccurate and caused unnecessary emotional stress. Fortunately the client was eventually able to embrace her own emotional journey and found acceptance in her own way.

COMPARISONS OUTSIDE OF RESIDENTIAL TREATMENT

Comparing progression is not just a residential-treatment issue. It happens "on the outs" as well, and it usually occurs on a larger level. People compare themselves to others as a way to validate or self-deprecate. For instance, people who attend twelve-step meetings might compare themselves to others based on days of sobriety or progression on step work. Another means of comparison, not surprisingly, is to assess material items. Who has his or her own place and who is still in sober living? Who has a car, a bank account, a job? Though all of these can be great things to celebrate when they're obtained, they also can be the basis for unhealthy comparisons.

Active addiction takes a lot away from an individual, and a goal for many is to regain those things. That goal-setting, though, has a tendency to become a race. It's as if there is a first-place prize for sobriety based on how fast you get your stuff back! When things move slowly, it can create a sense of inadequacy. People begin to feel ashamed of their life situations and try to force things to happen before they are ready. For instance, we've heard countless stories of people who move out of sober living and into their own apartment before they have the financial stability to do so, and they end up homeless within several months. Sometimes these people go back to sober living, but unfortunately, they usually fall into the victim role and begin using again.

It's important to remember that just because someone is doing well on paper does not mean she is living a healthy life. She might not be using, and she might have these things back in her life, but she could still engage in frequent unhealthy thought patterns or surround herself with unhealthy people. Days of sobriety and material possessions do not equal long-term sobriety. It's the things that are within and unseen that matter most.

It's Up to You!

Unfortunately, people will often use comparisons as reasons to give up. Whether it's leaving treatment or returning to using again, sometimes going back to when things were "easy" seems better than feeling inadequate. If someone accomplishes a milestone before you, it does not mean he is better than you are at sobriety; it simply means you're in different places on your own personal journeys. If you're having difficulty achieving a goal, have some conversations with a counselor or do some work on yourself to see what is holding you back and preventing you from progressing. No one gets anywhere just by hanging out. We call that "wood-working"—doing the bare minimum and not truly doing anything productive. Remember that your program is your program and no one else's. It is up to you to work it and up to you to maintain it—no one else can do that for you. If you aren't moving forward, it's your responsibility to discover why.

When you find yourself comparing yourself to others and feeling inadequate, it's your job to challenge it. It's also your responsibility to recognize what parts of your daily life might contribute to your unfair comparisons. Maybe you regularly go to a meeting where everyone has more money than you, or maybe you talk daily with your sister, whom you envy. It might be time to begin questioning your involvement with these influences. And that leads us to one of the biggest contributors of unfair comparison: social media.

SOCIAL MEDIA: MORE COMPLICATED THAN YOU THINK

Social media has become a major part of everyday life. When we stand in line or in a waiting room, it's rare not to see people scrolling on their phones. It's likely you do it, too! Social media sites have become a hub not only to receive news about our loved ones but also the world around us. People are constantly tweeting, uploading pictures, posting articles and videos—the list goes on—and we soak it all in. There is nothing inherently wrong with this. In many ways, social media does exactly what it is intended to do: It provides a convenient and fun way to keep in touch. It is not harmless, though, and it can contribute to those dangerous comparisons to which we all can fall victim. Even if you do not participate in social media, keep reading. You might be surprised by how it can affect you.

As we are scrolling, what do we tend to see? Highlights of significant life events, pictures with family and friends, announcements of marriages, births, and new purchases. What do these things have in common? They are all generally positive and happy. It's hard not to miss how many people are "liking" or responding to these posts. As we scroll, it's not uncommon to feel inadequate or envious. We might feel initially happy for our friends and acquaintances, but it's easy for our minds to wander. We might find ourselves thinking about how we don't have what they have and set unrealistic standards for ourselves.

What we've learned from our clients is that social media can be harmful in two primary ways. It can lead to victim thinking, and it can enable addictive behaviors.

Social Media and the Victim Role

Social media reminds people of everything they do not have thanks to their addiction. Because addiction strips away an individual's life, internally and externally, it can be depressing for a person to consistently scroll through updates of happy people with all the things that person has lost. That leads to unhealthy comparisons, which in turn can lead to adopting a victim mentality. For instance, browsing social media can evoke feelings of guilt, shame, and remorse over one's losses. It also can cause someone to engage in "what if" fantasizing about how her life could have been different if she had never become addicted. These thought patterns are not healthy or helpful. They can hinder a person's slow-but-steady progress down her own path because she is too busy focusing on someone else's path. If a person shames herself too frequently for her own journey, it is likely she will return to using.

Digital Bars and Trap Houses

Social media also can enable addictive behaviors if a client follows people who are in active addiction. Following people in active addiction means subjecting oneself to posts about use, pictures of people who are obviously drunk or high, and direct references to or pictures of the substances themselves.

Though no one can completely protect himself from these things, to actively engage with this type of content seems contradictory to the goals of sobriety. If someone is on a strict diet, would he walk into a bakery several times a day just to browse the sweets he's trying not to eat? When someone in recovery sees people engaging in substance use, he is likely to find himself entertaining thoughts about his own use. He might begin to romanticize his past use and focus only on the "good ol' days" of using. Constantly seeing others posting about these things, supposedly without any harm, can allow someone to forget just how much damage substance abuse caused. That's another form of dangerous comparison that can lead to using again.

STRONG OR SMART?

Right now you might be thinking, "Being affected by social media is just an excuse. Seeing that stuff makes you stronger!" And yes, there's some truth there. But let's really look closely. One goal of treatment is to assist clients in reframing their associations with "triggers" so they can exist in the world and not be constantly "triggered." Blaming use on being "triggered" by something negates your ability to make decisions. You're essentially saying that you are powerless over these things and have no choice but to use in the face of them. Well, we think you are more reasonable than that.

That said, we in no way encourage anyone to actively place himself into a potentially dangerous environment because he should be "strong enough" to handle it. This is just plain wrong, and to think otherwise is engaging in black-and-white thinking. To dismiss the negative impact some environments and relationships can have on a person is neglectful. If outside-world influences didn't exist, why would residential treatment centers exist? People in active addiction often need to remove themselves from their usual environments to allow themselves to reframe in a safe space. And people reframe at different paces, so to expect everyone to move at the same speed is yet another dangerous comparison.

HEALTHY SOCIAL MEDIA USE

So far we have basically villainized social media, but we do believe social media can be used in a healthy way. It's possible for people to use social media while still supporting their goals and keeping their focus. Here are several suggestions for doing just that:

1. Delete any unhealthy influencers from your friends list.

We are not just talking about the people with whom you used to use or who might post content about use. Think about removing the people to whom you consistently compare yourself. For instance, one client decided she needed to delete a lifelong friend of hers because seeing her friend's posts made her feel depressed and inadequate while she was in early recovery. It's perfectly okay to acknowledge that lessening unhealthy comparisons takes time, and if seeing consistent pictures of a friend's "perfect" life is difficult for you, consider taking a break from her social media for a while.

2. Recognize the reality.

It's easy to forget what social media truly is: a highlight reel. People post what they *want* other people to know about. Although there might be the occasional sad announcement, the majority of posts we see focus on good, positive events. What we are missing is the entire reality of a person's life. For instance, a person may post a happy picture with friends, but what we don't see are the daily struggles he experiences. Because we don't see those struggles, we make assumptions and comparisons. We rarely know the whole story behind these posts, and comparing ourselves to them is unfair to our own well-being.

3. Limit your time on social media.

Have you ever found yourself looking up from your phone or computer and realizing that more time went by than you thought? It's easy to get lost in the world of social media and neglect other responsibilities. Social media can be addictive in itself. More and more research suggests people can become dependent on social media. Also, the more time you're spending looking at other people's lives, the less time you're spending on yours. Set daily time limits for yourself, or even make it a reward to scroll once you've accomplished your tasks for the day.

4. Create a feed that inspires you.

Make the time you spend on social media worthwhile. Follow individuals or organizations that nourish you rather than deplete you. Fill your feeds with words of encouragement, inspirational posts, people you can relate to in a positive way, educational articles, cute puppy videos—whatever allows you to shut off your device and feel peaceful rather than anxious or depressed.

5. Be in the moment.

This might sound cliché, but its importance is undeniable. When we are engaged in social media, we are disengaged from the world around us. We are transporting ourselves to thousands of different locations within seconds and focusing heavily on the experiences of others. Reconnect with your own life. The options are endless for what you can do with it.

MOTIVATION RATHER THAN DEPRECATION

In this chapter, we have reviewed many ways people can engage in dangerous comparisons. As we wrap up, we want to acknowledge that comparison *can* be used for good. That's where role models, positive influences, and sponsors come in. There is a huge difference between wanting to be someone exactly (unrealistic, unhealthy) and wanting to pursue similar admirable qualities (realistic, healthy). We encourage people to seek out individuals they find relatable and inspirational in sobriety. By doing so, they can hopefully find the encouragement, guidance, and support they need to develop their own sense of self.

It's important to remember that you are enough, and you are worth it. When we compare ourselves to others, it can be difficult to remember those things. Use others' journeys to inform your own, but not dictate your own. Your journey will be your journey, but it is yours and only yours to take. It will look different from everyone else's, and that's exactly how it should be.

• • • LISA'S STORY • • •

Lisa entered treatment and initially appeared friendly, but her dark side began to show quickly. She frequently one-upped the other women in the facility and always had to have the better story. Lisa did not believe her drinking was a problem, saying things such as, "Well, it's not like I did *heroin.*" Lisa also appeared to be obsessed with her physical appearance, becoming angry if anything was out of place or imperfect.

Lisa was initially resistant to staff intervention, but eventually she began to open up. She revealed that, while growing up, her parents frequently compared her and her sisters. Her parents would comment on the girls' appearance and demean each one if she did not perform as well as the others. Lisa discovered that this obsession with comparison carried throughout her life.

Lisa realized that a main reason for her excessive alcohol use was to boost her confidence and feel okay with herself. She began to rely on alcohol because it provided her with a sense of security in the face of constant ridicule. During one group session, Lisa apologized to the group, stating that she realized she was so focused on others in the beginning because she was deeply ashamed of having gotten another DUI and facing the wrath of her parents.

Lisa compared herself to others in order to believe her problems weren't as bad. Once Lisa began to embrace her problems—and eventually herself—she began to make positive changes and care less about comparisons. Lisa decided to set boundaries with her parents and cease communication if they began to demean her. She graduated successfully from the program and is living a sober and less comparison-driven life.

FOR REFLECTION

- What are some dangerous comparisons that might be holding you back? Are there people you envy? Why?

_____

_____

_____

_____

_____

- How often do you use social media? When you do use it, which people and which kinds of posts make you feel good about yourself? Which make you feel inadequate or discouraged?

_____

_____

_____

_____

- Who are some people you view as role models—people you look up to for healthy comparisons and examples?

  _____

  _____

  _____

  _____

  _____

- Write down one negative comparison you commonly make about yourself. Now, reframe that thought in terms of how you're trying to change and grow. What is something positive you can say about yourself?

  _____

  _____

  _____

  _____

  _____

CHAPTER EIGHT

Managing Your Anger

Anger is one of the most misunderstood emotions. We vilify it and often see it as something negative. In some ways, this is for good reason. Anger can cause people to do some pretty crazy things, and it can definitely be a main driver for using substances. Take a moment to think about anger's role in your life. Have you ever done or said something out of anger that you now regret? Were you ever fueled by anger to drink or to use? For some of you, anger might have been a destructive force. For others, you might have been the target of someone else's anger and aggression. For many, it has been a mixture of both. Anger *can* be dangerous, but it does not have to be.

Many clients enter treatment and express a desire to work on their "anger problems." They see anger as the thing that needs to be fixed, and that isn't quite realistic. Anger is so much more than we tend to believe. In this chapter, we'll clear up the truth about anger and show you how you can embrace it and nurture it rather than push it away or allow it to control you.

HOOKED ON A FEELING

When it comes down to it, anger is simply an emotion. That's it. Anger is just like happiness, sadness, excitement, embarrassment…any other emotion. Everyone experiences anger, probably on a regular basis. The feeling can range from mild frustration to intense rage, depending on the individual and the situation. Feeling anger is actually very healthy. Anger, like any emotion, is the mind giving a cue on how to react to the world. To experience anger means you are human.

Feeling anger also helps us learn about ourselves—our morals, values, and boundaries. It can help us identify beliefs and thought patterns that aren't helpful for us. For instance, if you consistently find yourself bitter and angry whenever you talk to a certain family member, that's a cue that there might be something there to examine. What is it about that person that creates that feeling of anger? Is it something she does? The way he talks to you? What is your anger trying to tell you in that situation? Listen to it!

A SECONDARY EMOTION?

This leads us to address a common thing we hear in treatment: "Anger is a secondary emotion." This is a popular phrase, and it has some merit. But let's poke at it a bit. The primary intention of this phrase is to acknowledge that anger is often a reaction to another emotion that is less comfortable. As an example, here's a case study: A past client became furious when her father asked what she planned to do posttreatment. After processing, the client discovered that her anger came along with shame and confusion because she did not know her plan yet. She felt fear, too; she was afraid of life after treatment. Look at all those emotions! Shame, confusion, and fear—but she reacted with anger. She wasn't comfortable displaying her other emotions, because she believed they showed vulnerability. But delving into the other emotions that occur along with anger helps us get more in touch with our feelings. Yes, that probably sounds hokey, but it's true. Having an understanding and acceptance of your feelings is incredibly valuable, especially when pursuing sobriety.

Look at it this way: What was one appeal of using substances? Most clients would say not having to feel. In active addiction, you don't have to feel those uncomfortable emotions that nag at you. As you progressed in addiction, you could numb out the guilt you felt for stealing from your boyfriend, or the grief you felt over a dying family member. Here's the thing, though: Not dealing with emotions means not dealing with life. Without feeling your emotions, you aren't really living. You're shutting out a major piece of the human experience.

Bottling emotions in sobriety is similar to numbing them in active addiction. Pretending they don't exist and wearing a mask of contentedness hinders you from the growth necessary to truly move forward. If you're not allowing yourself to be aware of your emotions, you cannot process them and you cannot learn from them. Not learning means you are remaining stagnant. Remaining stagnant means that eventually something will come along that challenges you, and because you haven't developed coping skills for the emotions you've spent so much time bottling, you won't know how to deal with it. When you don't know how to deal with something, you resort to what you *do* know: returning to using substances.

So where does anger fit in? Anger itself is an emotion like any other emotion. But demoting anger to being purely a "secondary emotion" can have some troubling consequences. Dealing with feelings of shame, guilt, fear, and sadness without also addressing anger is an incomplete solution. We can't just pretend the anger is not there—that's just bottling. While we can acknowledge that a lot of emotions reside underneath anger, let's not take away anger's validity.

As we said before, anger can be scary. But if it's something we naturally *should* feel, why are we constantly receiving messages that anger is a bad thing? Why do things like anger-management courses exist? It's all because of a common misconception—confusing *anger* with *aggression*.

EMOTIONS VERSUS BEHAVIORS

It's easy to get anger and aggression mixed up. In fact, many people use the words interchangeably. They are very different, though, and that's an important thing to recognize. Anger is an emotion. It's something we feel and experience within ourselves. Aggression, meanwhile, is a behavior. Aggression is the hostile, forceful, sometimes violent behavior that can result from anger. This is where people get in trouble. There is nothing wrong with feeling anger, but it is detrimental to act out in aggression.

It can be difficult to grasp that anger can be responded to in a different way. For many, aggression is the natural response to anger. Becoming aggressive, whether verbally, physically, or both, is how you get the point across that you are angry. Isn't that just nature? Actually, no. Research shows that aggression is a learned response.

Think about what you learned about anger while growing up around your family, friends, people at school, and people in your community. How would your family communicate anger to one another? Would it be a stern but calm conversation or a screaming match? When your friends hurt your feelings, did you calmly talk about your feelings or did you threaten to fight them, or even actually hit them? Community violence is also common for some in both childhood and adulthood when individuals live in dangerous areas where drugs and gangs are rampant.

Think back to your childhood. Did you realize at some point that if you became aggressive, you got your way? Many people have learned, whether as children or adults, how they can utilize their anger and aggression to manipulate others. They use rage and violence to get their way. While in active addiction, a person learns he can use aggression to get what he wants. Like any learned behavior, that then can continue into sobriety. Many clients struggle with not resorting to aggression when they are challenged, because it has become their first go-to.

That leads us to "venting." When we talk about anger management, many people like to tout certain coping skills such as "punching a pillow," "hitting a punching bag," "hitting a wall," "smashing something," and so on. People tend to think that because the aggression isn't directed toward other people, it's okay. This type of "coping" actually has been shown through research not to be helpful. In fact, it has been shown to make people *more* aggressive. That sort of "coping" only reinforces aggressive behavior. If, after becoming angry, you haul off and punch a pillow for five minutes, you are still engaging in aggression as a way to express what you're feeling. And where is the processing? There is no discussion and little learning from the experience. Addressing anger with aggression simply leads to more aggression.

So when someone says she wants to address her "anger" issues, she is probably referring to her "aggression" issues. She wants to learn how to cope with anger so she does not blow up in an aggressive rage. For some, this can be very difficult. Many people have relied on aggression to get through life. They wear it like a mask that is hard to take off. It is possible, though. We've seen plenty of the "angriest" clients work hard and develop much healthier ways of coping with their emotions. Even if anger is not an "issue" for you, we still encourage you to review our suggestions and see if there are places where you can make improvements.

Awareness and Anger

When working on modifying anger responses, most of it boils down to awareness. If you are struggling with aggression, here are some things to pay attention to:

1. What makes you angry?

It's time to take inventory of what specifically creates feelings of anger within you. What happens throughout your day that incites feelings of anger—and consequently an aggressive response? Don't overthink this, and recognize that things will clock in at different "levels." One thing might make you mildly annoyed, while another might have you furious. Acknowledge *all* of it. The little things matter just as much as the big things, especially because they often add up. Start taking note (seriously, write them down!) of the things that irritate you throughout the day. Over time, you will begin to notice patterns.

2. What are your cues?

Start to get in touch with yourself. As you identify the things that cause your anger, also pay attention to what's happening within you when you're angry. There are four different areas to be aware of:

    a. Physical: heavy breathing, increased heart rate, tightness in chest and/or stomach, face becoming flushed

    b. Behavioral: squinting eyes, snarling, clenching fists, cracking knuckles, raising voice

    c. Emotional: feeling disrespected, scared, disappointed, embarrassed

    d. Cognitive: irrational thought patterns, violent or aggressive thoughts, negative self-talk

Though it can be challenging, taking time to note how your body is responding in these areas during a moment of anger can be very helpful. When you begin to identify your cues, you can de-escalate yourself before things get out of hand. You also might begin to notice that your anger levels are "rising" as the day goes on. This is why taking note of the little things is so important in step one! If at midday you notice your physical and behavioral cues are starting to kick in, you can start implementing other coping skills to calm down before you really get going.

3. What works for you?

Here's where the real work comes in. We are not going to give you a nice little list of coping mechanisms for anger and guarantee success if you use them. The truth is it will be trial and error. You are going to need to try different things multiple times and evaluate how well each works for you. In fact, you might even need different coping mechanisms for different situations. Removing yourself from a situation might help during an argument with a parent, but that's not exactly possible when you're stuck in traffic. Here are some places to start, though.

    a. Deep breathing exercises: This could be counting to certain numbers, focusing intently on your breathing, deliberately breathing in and out at a certain pace, etc. Implementing this when you begin to recognize those physical cues can help halt them from intensifying.

b. Utilize personal mantras or soothing self-talk: Many clients see value in this technique. When you begin to feel those cues, start self-soothing through mantras or positive affirmation. Repeating something like "You are calm" or "Just breathe; you're okay" can help instill a sense of calm.

c. Challenge any self-defeating thoughts: Take note of those cognitive cues. What are some things going through your mind? Can any of it possibly be challenged or altered to create a healthier mind-set? Start taking note of these things and consider adopting alternate views.

d. Regularly engage in hobbies and self-care: This is more of a long-term coping mechanism, and that's what makes it important. By regularly engaging in activities you find soothing and enjoyable, you are more likely to feel less stressed. A lowered state of stress can mean feeling less reactive to anger-inducing situations. It's like a car. If you don't take care of it, eventually it will clunk out on the highway. If you perform regular maintenance, it is more likely you'll have smoother sailing.

There are dozens of suggestions for how to cope with anger outside of aggression. We highly encourage you to research and try as many as possible. Maybe even consider reaching out to a mental-health professional. The more tools you have, the more prepared you are! We are going to discuss one more, though, and it's a big one. It's less of a coping skill and more of a life skill, and it can improve many areas of your life if mastered.

ASSERTIVENESS

When it comes to anger and aggressiveness, it's important to acknowledge the importance of effective communication. Being able to respond to conflict, no matter how frustrating, without aggression is an important skill to learn. We focus heavily on better communication in our program because we believe it is so important. When clients develop more effective ways of speaking their minds, they find that their relationships improve and so does their quality of life.

In general, there are four main communication styles. In the explanations below, we will provide an example based on one scenario: You're at the grocery store and the cashier rings up your order incorrectly. As he hands you your receipt, you notice the mistake. Your response is:

1. Passive: A person with a passive communication style tends to avoid any forms of conflict, whether genuine or perceived. He will have difficulty expressing his thoughts or feelings and often will choose to say nothing at all. He also might unnecessarily apologize and/or immediately agree with a differing opinion. This type of communication often creates resentments and bitterness due to true emotions being bottled and going unacknowledged. Example: "Oh, that's...um...okay, thank you."

2. Aggressive: Aggressive communication styles are loud, forceful, and accusatory. A person with this style of speaking will share her feelings and opinions in a way that directly belittles others. She might even use physical aggression or intimidation to get her point across, such as slamming down a fist or waving her arms as she speaks. People who adopt this style are continuously fueling that aggressive behavior and pushing others away with it. Example: "Are you kidding me? I can't believe you. This is a whole $15 off from what it should be! Are you stupid?"

3. Passive-Aggressive: A passive-aggressive style is evident through indirect and sarcastic comments. This person wants to avoid conflict yet still wants to have his say. Therefore, he chooses to address his opinions and feelings in ways that aren't entirely clear and might even be contradictory. For instance, he might smile while expressing disgust. Similar to passivity, these individuals tend to develop resentments and can alienate themselves due to their excessive sarcasm and inability to clearly express themselves. Example: "Huh...I mean, sure, I guess I can pay a whole $15 more. Like I'm just rolling in cash right now, buddy."

4. Assertive: A person with an assertive communication style is able to calmly express her opinions and concerns in a way that is direct. She is comfortable sharing her feelings in relation to something and does not use accusatory statements. Listening is also a trait of assertive communication,

as it takes into account the opinion and response of the other person. Individuals who adopt this style experience connectedness and build understanding with others. Their conversations are less anger-inducing due to the healthy expression of emotion. Example: "Excuse me…it actually said another price on the display. It appears to be more on my receipt. Do you think you could look at that for me and change it? I would appreciate it!"

As you look at these different communication styles, which one do you align with the most? If it's not assertive, it's time to start making some changes. Communicating more effectively will assist you with managing anger and decreasing aggression. When people are clearly expressing emotions and thoughts and engaging in true discussion, there is less room for argument and accusation. Even if one person is assertive and the other is not, the assertive individual has confidence in his or her own words and can cope with any uncomfortable feelings that arise from the conversation. Learning to communicate in an assertive fashion is an important piece not only of anger management, but also of life. Think about your relationships and how these communication styles might be present within them. Now think about what it might be like if everyone clearly and calmly expressed themselves in a direct and non-accusatory manner.

You're probably thinking, *Ha! Like that will ever happen!* Okay, fair enough. It's difficult for people to respond with assertiveness 100 percent of the time. That's because it's not based on impulsive and emotional decision-making. Look at the other styles. All of those fall in line with some sort of flight-or-fight response—are you going to back down, fight it, or a little of both? That's primal reasoning right there, and we believe we are all better than that.

We encourage all our clients (and ourselves!) to learn to communicate more assertively. When the majority of the community begins to adopt this style, the therapeutic process goes much more smoothly, and there is less conflict. Clients are receptive to one another and can acknowledge the differing opinions amongst them without turmoil. This isn't a fairy-tale world, we promise. This is real life built on communicating like humans, not animals.

ANGER AND REAL LIFE

One thing to remember is that it is unlikely you will handle your anger 100 percent correctly 100 percent of the time, and that's okay. There will be some days when you bottle it and others when it explodes all over the place. The goal here is for consistency. Are you consistently feeling calm and capable of coping with your uncomfortable emotions? Do you feel like you are in control of how you handle them rather than responding like a puppet to their whims? Consistency is definitely key here, because beating yourself up for not doing it perfectly will only set you back.

And obviously you will still feel anger. Don't forget that whole "anger is natural and necessary" thing we talked about at the beginning of this chapter. Embracing anger as another emotion, rather than one to fear or feel controlled by, will help you utilize those coping skills. Learning new and more effective ways to communicate also will assist with your ability to have tough conversations without blowing up and will give you a way to express thoughts and feelings healthfully rather than bottling them.

If coping with anger and aggression is something you struggle with, we hope some of the insights in this chapter are helpful to you. Like everything else in this book, the concepts presented here are not magic, and they will take work to develop. We believe everyone can choose to embrace a calmer state of mind, and we hope that is true for you!

• • • RICK'S STORY • • •

Rick entered treatment angry. He would blow up at other clients for minor incidents and at staff for not allowing him special privileges. When addressed, Rick would say, "It's just who I am. I was born angry. I came out of the womb swinging, and that's how I'll go out."

Clients and staff tried to connect with Rick, but it would go only so far before he would storm off, muttering obscenities. Rick was never violent, but his aggression came out through his words and expressions. He would become especially angry when discussing his wife, who had given him an ultimatum to get help or get out. Rick shared stories of them arguing and told how he used drugs to calm himself down.

Rick was not open to the idea of finding other coping methods; he believed he needed heroin to remain calm. He thought this because of his deep belief that he was "just an angry person." Despite multiple staff and client interventions, Rick was resistant to making changes.

One day, when his counselor addressed him, Rick became angry and punched a hole in the wall. Rick was discharged immediately due to violent behavior. We hope he was able to eventually see the truth and get help.

FOR REFLECTION

- How do you act when you feel angry? Do you feel your coping mechanisms are healthy?

_____

_____

_____

_____

_____

- Which communication style (passive, aggressive, passive-aggressive, assertive) best describes how you interact with others? Is there anything you would like to change about your communication style?

_____

_____

_____

_____

_____

- What sorts of situations or circumstances tend to make you angry? What are the roots of your anger in those instances?

  _____

  _____

  _____

  _____

  _____

CHAPTER NINE

Forgiving Yourself and Others

When clients come into our facility, we create an individualized treatment plan that covers the issues each client needs to address. One of the most common goals we hear is the desire to mend the bridges burned with family, friends, significant others, and children during active addiction.

When people enter into sobriety, one of the first major hurdles they experience is the flood of emotions smacking them in the face. They begin to remember what they've done in active addiction, and they feel guilt, shame, anger—all the uncomfortable emotions they spent years numbing. The thought of asking for forgiveness feels overwhelming, and they wonder if they can ever regain the trust of their loved ones.

It's also likely that they will begin remembering all the terrible things other people have done to them. They play those situations through their heads and build resentment toward the individuals in question. At that point, they might even reject the concept of forgiveness. It might feel out of reach or impossible to forgive or to be forgiven.

One reason forgiveness feels like such a big deal is because it's misunderstood. When we see forgiveness for what it really is, it begins to feel more possible.

Let's be upfront right now: This chapter will not give you a list of steps or any easy solutions to forgiveness. It will not provide a guide to follow in order to forgive. We don't believe that is realistic. Instead, we are going to challenge some common ideas about forgiveness and present some thinking points to help set you on the path toward peace.

Forgiveness Is Complicated

The most common misconception about forgiveness is that it's a linear process. The way forgiveness is typically presented goes something like this: Bad thing happens; bad feelings ensue; dramatic moment of forgiveness occurs; happiness abounds. The relationship is mended, and all is well forever and ever. If that sounds too good to be true, that's because it is. It's completely unrealistic, which is why forgiveness feels so unattainable. The truth is, forgiveness is complicated. But it *is* doable.

Forgiveness does not follow a set path. It will have twists and turns, ups and downs. Every situation that involves forgiveness will look different and have its own challenges. We also need to take into account the fact that humans are involved, so the process of forgiveness is going to depend on the people in the mix and the emotions and perceptions they have wrapped up in the situation. The severity of the action also needs to be considered. Forgiveness for accidentally bumping someone in line will look significantly different from forgiveness for stealing someone's life savings and spending it on drugs. There are a lot of different factors, so expecting forgiveness to be a straightforward path is setting yourself up for failure.

Holding on to baseless expectations can lead to feelings of anger or resentment. Even worse, the unmet expectations can bring about a victim mentality, which all too easily can turn into using again. For instance, a lot of people in early sobriety develop a belief that, because they are sober, their loved ones will forgive them instantly. But embracing a life without substances does not suddenly erase years of stealing, lying, and fighting. That disconnect can build a foundation of dysfunction rather than one of healing.

I Want It, and I Want It NOW!

Instant gratification is a common issue not only for those who have lived in active addiction, but for humans in general. We live in an age when receiving things quickly is the norm. Things like high-speed Internet and two-day shipping have us accustomed to getting what we want as soon as it comes to mind.

Addiction takes that desire to another level. When you're dependent on a substance, you're subject to its demands. When it wants you to have it, it wants you to have it *now*, and you will feel terrible until you can get it. Whether it's terrible physically, emotionally, or both, you will do anything you can, as fast as you can, to get that next fix. That's the nature of addiction, and it makes the expectation of instant gratification become a default.

When the substance is taken out of the picture, the need for instant gratification does not go with it. Many clients enter treatment with a sense of entitlement that when they want something, they should be able to obtain it immediately. Most programs have processes in place to help with this, and they're usually met with resistance or frustration. Though the reaction is understandable, it is important to challenge that "I want it now" mind-set. That way of thinking is directly tied to addictive thinking, and there is little benefit in holding onto mentalities from active addiction. The obvious truth is that not everything can happen all at once, and sometimes we need to wait for things.

How does this relate to forgiveness? As we've discussed, forgiveness is complicated because humans are involved. That means forgiveness might not progress on the timeline you have in mind. You might *want* the forgiveness of your father, but maybe he needs more time to heal. You might *want* to stop obsessing over your ex-boyfriend cheating on you, but perhaps there are details you need to process before you can lessen the burden on your mind. And even when you've moved totally into the forgiveness stage, it doesn't mean that everything is suddenly all better. There will still be challenges along the way.

You might become frustrated because you want the pain to end. You just want things to go back to "normal"—the way things were before. That's okay, and, if anything, that *is* normal. Real normalcy—or reality—is being able to accept life on its timeline, not yours. Let's reflect on chapter three, when we talked about trusting the process. Forgiveness is a perfect example of how trusting the process is necessary. When you are on the road to forgiveness, there will be days when it feels endless or like you're going in circles. There will be times when you want to give up, and there might even be days when you want to use to numb the pain. This is when challenging the need for instant gratification and trusting the process is so essential.

FORGIVE AND FORGET?

Contrary to popular belief, the old saying "forgive and forget" is not great advice. In fact, it's quite dangerous. Talk about unrealistic expectations! Unfortunately, we cannot simply forget things because we want to, especially if they were significantly impactful to our lives. Also, why *should* we forget? Forgetting does not simply mean forgetting about an event, but also forgetting the valuable lessons that event could provide us. Our experiences and memories are what shape us. They inform our actions and contribute to our windows of perception. When we hurt someone or someone hurts us, we make modifications to our behavior to prevent that from happening again. We need to accept this as part of life rather than reject it and pretend things never occurred.

"Forgive and forget" is also dangerous because it discredits the impact of an action. It suggests that everything hurtful that happens to us, or that we do to someone else, simply can be swept under the rug. If we tell ourselves that this should be the reality, how will we feel about ourselves when it isn't? We might feel inadequate or like something is "wrong" with us. Sometimes "forgive and forget" is even used to shame someone who is struggling to forgive or who has not been forgiven. Has someone ever said something to you along the lines of, "You just need to forgive, forget, and move on," with a hint of exasperation? The implication is that forgiving and forgetting is the standard, and if you cannot live up to this standard, then you're doing it wrong.

In reality what you need to forget is that phrase! If you want to truly pursue forgiveness, instead of "forgive and forget," try embracing a new idea: "Forgive and accept."

FORGIVE AND ACCEPT

Acceptance is essential to the forgiveness cycle because it sets a foundation for being open to possibilities. Many people seek forgiveness because they want things to go back to the way they were before. The truth is, that's impossible. The event has changed things on some level, and although forgiveness is possible, the relationship returning to its previous state is not. It's like a scar—the skin heals, but part of it is changed.

Now, let's not jump straight to black-and-white thinking and see this as negative. This is, yet again, where trusting the process comes in. People in recovery need to trust that these moments of change are for the better and they can grow and develop from them regardless of the outcome. The relationship could become stronger, or it could end. Or possibly it could land somewhere in between.

Trying to force forgiveness in order to force a relationship to remain the same is allowing that control monster to come out. Forgiveness does not always mean that a person will remain in your life. In fact, you might be in the process of forgiving someone—or being forgiven by someone—who has been out of your life for quite a while.

Accepting what happened as part of your story is also necessary for forgiveness. It's not easy, but forgiveness isn't possible if we cannot enter into a state of acceptance over the event in question. You might be wondering how you can possibly accept what you've done or what has been done to you. That is a totally valid question, and the truth is that it will take a lot of work. Back to the point about instant gratification: The most important things rarely happen quickly.

A CHAPTER, NOT THE WHOLE STORY

One of the most vital things for you to remember is that your life in active addiction is not your entire story; it is merely a chapter. It's easy to fall into the victim role when we begin to label ourselves and define our lives by the shameful things we've done or the horrible things that have happened to us.

In order to begin lessening the burden of these events, we need to look at them in different ways. Take a minute to think about how you currently view a situation in your life where forgiveness is needed. What types of words surround it? What types of attitudes or beliefs? What roadblocks are you noticing?

For instance, let's say you feel guilty for wrecking your mother's car while in active addiction. Look at that first feeling word: *guilty*. What other words come with that? *Ashamed* maybe? *Stupid, careless, disappointing, scary, angry*—these are all possibilities. Notice how much negative weight these words hold. Let's say you view this event as the one that caused your mother to no longer trust you, the moment she became fully aware of how serious and dangerous your substance use had become. This is when the arguments started and she began hiding not only her keys from you but her other valuables as well. It was a major tipping point, and one you beat yourself up for daily.

How can you view this in a way that fosters forgiveness? Well, to start simply, you can tell yourself the event was beneficial in the long run because it helped you realize the need for treatment. Or perhaps you can develop a sense of gratitude that you did not hurt yourself or someone else in the crash. You can begin to process through your feelings of anger and disappointment in yourself and recognize that your past actions do not define your current self. When it comes to your mom, you can accept that her journey through forgiveness is her own, and she will travel it in her own time. You can recognize that certain privileges might be absent for a while and take ownership of the consequences of your actions. You can accept that your mom might not trust you for a while—or maybe ever again—and you can live with that.

Do you see the reframing happening here? This is related to what's called "narrative therapy," a counseling theory and style in which focus is placed on our stories and how we view them. Narrative therapy allows us to revisit past events and tell their stories in alternative ways that might be healthier. When you are in the process of forgiving, you are essentially confronting a story you revisit again and again in a way that is painful. Taking time to rewrite that chapter in some way and change its language can assist you in moving forward.

No one else can do this for you, though. It's up to you to begin rewriting those stories and reframing their impact on you. It's a process that might take days, weeks, months, or years—and that's okay. Remember: Your timeline is your timeline—no one else's.

FORGIVENESS IS FOR YOU

When it comes to forgiveness, it's important to remember that it is not for anyone but yourself. That might sound confusing, because we're generally raised to believe that forgiveness is a process for others, whether it is granting forgiveness *to someone* or gaining forgiveness *from someone*. In the grand scheme, though, forgiveness has nothing to do with that "someone" and everything to do with you.

Let's revisit the aforementioned situation with Mom. Let's say she forgave you prior to doing any of that narrative work. Would it have really lessened the feelings of guilt you had or the disappointment you felt in yourself? Think about it. When someone forgives you for something you still feel terrible about, do you really feel better? Maybe temporarily, but in the long run, it's unlikely. Clients in treatment experience this all the time. They wait and wait for that forgiveness and then feel confused when they don't feel better for having received it.

And consider this: What about situations in which a person who wronged you has died, or you have no way to contact him or her? If you believe forgiveness is all about that other person—not about yourself—then forgiveness would be impossible in many uncontrollable circumstances. That's the danger of viewing forgiveness as an external process, something that needs to be outwardly granted or received. Unless words are exchanged, it's basically meaningless, right? Wrong.

Fortunately forgiveness doesn't work that way. Forgiveness is a purely internal process. It is something that each person can gain or grant without another person involved. In fact, to forgive independently gives you a sense of agency and control over your life. It empowers you to heal and keep writing your chapters without waiting for someone to give you permission. No one can heal you, just as you can't heal others. It has to happen within.

Now, we aren't saying it isn't nice to be able to have that forgiveness conversation with another person and possibly find a resolution. And we definitely aren't saying you should never grant or ask for forgiveness. If it's possible and healthy, those conversations are immensely beneficial. What we are saying, though, is that more is needed for true healing, and healing is possible without other people involved.

This is especially important for people who have abusive individuals in their lives. Reconnecting with someone who could cause you emotional and/or physical harm might not be healthy for the sake of forgiveness. There are so many other ways to find closure rather than placing yourself in an unsafe situation.

FORGIVENESS IS A CHOICE

Forgiveness truly is a choice. There has to be a willingness and a desire to forgive or to be forgiven. Without that will and motivation, the process will be an empty one. Don't pursue forgiveness because you believe you "should." Do it because you recognize that you deserve to heal. Acknowledge that, regardless of what you have done or what has been done to you, forgiveness is possible.

Don't forget to be gentle with yourself in the process and recognize that healing, as with any physical wound, takes time. Eventually you will see it as merely another chapter in the intricate story of your life.

• • • MEGAN'S STORY • • •

Megan entered our program bitter and angry. She had deep resentment toward many people in her life, including her family and ex-boyfriend. Megan expressed hatred toward these individuals because they were abusive and introduced her to drugs. Megan did not understand how forgiveness could even be possible. These people had done horrible things to her, and some of them weren't even alive anymore. For a while Megan stood firm in her belief that her family and ex did not deserve forgiveness. Why should she grant forgiveness, something she viewed as sacred, to people who hurt her so deeply?

The community sympathized with Megan, and some even agreed that she should hold onto those resentments based on the stories she told. As Megan progressed through the program, though, she began to recognize that some of her beliefs about forgiveness weren't entirely helpful. In fact, she saw them as a hindrance in many ways. She learned that she was also applying those beliefs toward herself, which made it difficult for her to move forward. Megan recognized that she felt ashamed of many things she did in active addiction and had a difficult time forgiving herself because she did not feel she deserved it.

Through her work in the program, Megan began to develop new beliefs about forgiveness. Megan forgave herself for her wrongdoings and identified reasons she deserved that forgiveness. She also forgave her family and ex-boyfriend through a ceremony she did with her fellow clients. Megan recognized that she needed to remain distant from these people, but she could move forward in life without allowing her resentments to hinder her. Megan graduated from the program feeling, as she said, "lighter" and with a more positive outlook on life.

For Reflection

- Why do you think forgiveness is a process and not just a simple action?

- Recall a time when you forgave someone. Did you tell the person, or was the process more internal? How did you feel once you'd granted that forgiveness?

- How do you feel about the phrase "forgive and forget"? What are some good things that could come of forgiving someone without forgetting the original situation?

- What is something in your life for which you would like forgiveness? What would it mean to you to be forgiven?

_____

_____

_____

_____

_____

CHAPTER TEN

Dealing with Death

As we've mentioned several times, one of the biggest challenges for people in early recovery is the return of emotions. After years of being masked by substances, emotions return with full force in sobriety, and they can feel overwhelming. Even daily, regular feelings can seem difficult to bear to someone who has avoided them for a long period of time. In the first few days of sobriety, some clients even worry that they're suffering from mental illness because their emotions are such a roller-coaster ride. With time, processing, and support, however, people "level out" and realize it's simply part of being sober—feeling things again, all the time.

Within this process comes another challenge: remembering painful events from the past. Clients might begin to dwell on events about which they were originally apathetic because of their use. Things that happened years ago are being felt and processed as if they happened yesterday. An especially difficult piece of that puzzle is recognizing the death and loss clients experienced (or avoided experiencing) while in active addiction. When many clients become sober, it begins to sink in that certain family members and friends are no longer alive. This is a very hard realization, and it requires effort to work through.

Other clients, meanwhile, might experience the death of a friend or loved one while in treatment. That shock can become an excuse for leaving treatment and returning to active addiction, but it doesn't have to be.

An unfortunate reality is that life does not pause because you decide to pursue sobriety; life does not work on our individual timelines. Though it would be wonderful for things to halt until you become comfortable in sobriety and develop lots of new coping skills and perspectives, it doesn't work that way. Things will continue happening around you, and you will have to deal with them in real time.

Though death can be scary, it is also a natural process of life. It's inevitable for all of us. It's extremely difficult (and not entirely realistic) for us to become "comfortable" with death. What we can do, though, is begin to view it in a way that nurtures us rather than depletes us. As with most things, the way we choose to view death determines the way it affects us. Let's explore some ideas about death that might help reframe our thoughts.

GUILT, SHAME, AND SELF-DEFEAT

Clients often express a lot of guilt, shame, and self-defeat in reaction to death. There are multiple reasons for this: They were under the influence during the death, they have a history of using with the person who has died, they missed someone's final days because of using, and so on. Because emotions are in abundance, so are self-defeating thoughts. The emotions present during a time of loss, or even when remembering loss, can create thought patterns that are not helpful—or even true. Let's take a look at some common reactions to loss.

"I SHOULD HAVE BEEN AROUND MORE, AND NOW HE'S GONE."

When a person experiences a painful loss, one of her first reactions is regretting the time she did not spend with the person. She thinks to herself, *I should have called more...I should have visited more...I should have spent more time with him.* This is especially difficult for people who are newly sober, because the time they did not spend with their loved one was usually spent getting drunk or high. They also realize the time they *did* spend with that person was usually when they were under the influence. This is a painful thing to acknowledge and is difficult to accept.

The obvious truth is that we cannot change the past, but we can use it as inspiration to change the future. Sure, you might believe you should have spent more time with someone, but you didn't. There is the hard reality. You do not need to leave it there, though. If you are beating yourself up for not spending proper time with people in the past, moments like this can help you realize where to re-prioritize. You already have made the decision to pursue sobriety, and that is an amazing step in itself. Now you also can think about other ways you can prioritize the important people in your life and what you can do differently moving forward.

"She died of an overdose, and I was the one who introduced her to drugs."

Clients often struggle with news of an overdose, especially if they introduced that person to drugs. Many clients find themselves responsible for such deaths. A client in this situation often will wonder: *Why did that person have to die? Why not me? Do I even deserve to be in treatment right now if I'm the reason someone died from this stuff?* These types of thoughts can be very dangerous, and it's important to see the reality. We are not suggesting that people ignore the influence they've had on others. We are promoters of accountability and taking ownership of actions. But the key word there is "influence."

There is a major difference between recognizing oneself as an *influence* and seeing oneself as a *cause*. Every one of us has influence on others in some way. Humans are social beings who take cues from their surroundings—it's just part of our nature. Introducing someone to drugs makes you an *influence*, but humans have the ability to make their own decisions. If a person chose to use the drugs you introduced him to, that was his choice. This might be hard to accept, but unless you somehow invented a mind-control device and decided *for* that person to do the drug, you were not the cause. Being able to distinguish the differences between influence and cause will allow you to see things more clearly and hopefully lessen those feelings of guilt.

"I WAS SO MESSED UP AT THE FUNERAL. I DON'T EVEN
REMEMBER IT." OR, "I WAS SO MESSED UP, I DIDN'T EVEN
MAKE IT TO THE FUNERAL."

Funerals are interesting things. They're a time for remembrance, celebration of life, and grief over death. Many view funerals as a time of "closure," believing that attending the funeral will provide a sense of peace with the death. Many clients express how they don't feel "closure" over a death because they were under the influence during the funeral or didn't attend at all. Again, this is a matter of perception. Funerals are not magic, and most of the time, they do not provide closure for the people who attend. The pain of that loss is still there, and it will take more than an event to bring that sense of peace. Closure is found through time, not in a singular moment.

Clients also struggle with feeling shame over missing a funeral or not being sober while in attendance. They believe it was disrespectful to the person who died, and there is no way they can make it up to that person. Regret over past actions is a natural part of early sobriety and, honestly, of life in general. But remember: Healing and forgiveness can be found even if a person is no longer around. It's up to you to determine how you can forgive yourself and move forward. Pursuing sobriety can be a way to honor a deceased loved one. It can be a major motivation for remaining sober and bettering one's life.

EXPERIENCING AND DEALING WITH GRIEF

The most common question we receive when clients are dealing with grief and loss is, "How do I get through this?" Unfortunately they want something that doesn't exist: an easy solution to their pain. They don't want to feel the discomfort and agony of a loss. This makes sense because their previous way of dealing with things *was* easy, and it numbed them well. But now, those pesky emotions are back.

Many clients actually have become desensitized to death. A lifestyle of addiction often means experiencing frequent loss, and when you experience something so frequently, it's easy to become indifferent to it. An attitude of indifference carries over into sobriety, and that's not healthy. It's important to learn how to embrace those feelings and allow yourself to mourn. Don't disregard death and the emotions associated with it just because it's common, and don't bottle emotions just because they are uncomfortable. When you refuse to feel that hurt, you are wearing a mask and choosing to continue behaviors associated with addiction. Numbing your emotions is something you did in active addiction, and it will not serve you in sobriety.

Another issue we see is on the other end of the spectrum: overprocessing a death from the past because it was not fully processed when it actually occurred. Some people in treatment might be mourning a death anywhere from a year to fifteen years prior. As a person enters sobriety, he remembers and recognizes those losses and might feel them as if they happened recently. That emotional reaction can feel almost crippling. Often people will obsess over these losses and find it difficult to focus on anything else. This is when an individual needs help in reframing the self-defeating thoughts that occur in conjunction with extreme grief.

Death and grief cannot be ignored, but they should not be obsessed over. The challenge is finding a balance. There are several theories that suggest how people can process death in a healthy way, and we will briefly discuss two primary views here: the five stages of grief and the theory of meaning reconstruction. It's important to note that there is no one, definitive way to handle grief.

THE FIVE STAGES OF GRIEF

In 1969 Elisabeth Kübler-Ross published *On Death and Dying*, which introduced five stages that many people might encounter when reacting to a death:

1. Denial and isolation: In reaction to death, a person may deny the reality of the situation. Masking and bottling of emotions also might occur in this stage.

2. Anger: The overwhelming emotions associated with the loss are channeled into feelings of anger and blame. This is often due to feeling vulnerable or weak in the face of loss.

3. Bargaining: In this stage, the individual strives to regain control though bargaining—"If we do this, maybe it won't happen"—or contemplation of alternate possibilities—"If only we'd gone to the doctor sooner."

4. Depression: The individual experiences feelings of sadness, regret, shame, and other emotions in reaction to the loss.

5. Acceptance: The individual feels a sense of calm and peace in reaction to the loss. This does not necessarily mean happiness or indifference.

Kübler-Ross proposed that people in mourning will experience these stages at different intensities, in different orders, and at different lengths of time. Some people might even skip stages and not experience them at all. There is no timeline for each stage, and people can move back and forth between the stages before eventually coming to terms with the loss and feeling acceptance.

Many people find guidance and hope in Kübler-Ross's theory and the materials associated with it. The acknowledgment that experiencing a range of emotions and reactions to grief can help it feel more "normal."

MEANING RECONSTRUCTION

Another common theory and practice in grief work is meaning reconstruction. The thought behind this approach is that experiencing a loss can be a significant part of someone's story. It can challenge a person's beliefs about the world and his or her place in it, especially when a loss is particularly painful. By processing the meaning and impact a loss has upon someone's life and what it means for his or her story, a person can create a sense of peace.

Many clients enjoy reading the book *Man's Search for Meaning* by Viktor Frankl, which details his experience in a concentration camp during World War II. Frankl pioneers the idea of meaning-making by discussing how different individuals within the camp viewed being there and what meaning they placed upon it. It's an emotional read, but one that helps put things into perspective.

It can be very helpful for clients to reconstruct the meaning they attribute to different events in their lives, loss being one of them. For instance, if a client views the death of a childhood friend as a tragedy that created a belief that the world is unfair and dangerous, she can reconstruct those views. She can begin to see that event as one that taught her she can be strong; she can see the loss as something that brought her family together or led her to a new and even more nurturing friendship. When it comes down to it, you are the one who decides what meaning, significance, and outcome you place upon an event. These things can break you down or continue to mold you. Events are merely parts of your personal story, and you're the one who decides how that story will be written.

REMEMBERING REALITY

No matter how you decide to deal with grief, it's important to remember how necessary it is to actually deal with it, not just ignore it and hope it goes away. As we've discussed, loss can have a large impact on our lives, but it's ultimately up to us what type of impact that is. Will it be something that destroys or something that inspires growth?

It's totally normal to feel powerless in the face of death, but the truth is that we have more control than we might realize. It's entirely in your power to decide how you will continue to live and who you will be. The loss of another's life does not have to be the loss of yours. Keep yourself healthy, surround yourself with support, and you can come out stronger.

• • • JASON'S STORY • • •

Jason entered treatment after fifteen years of active addiction. Jason had brief periods of sobriety but ultimately would begin using again. In his first session, Jason cited the death of his father as the most impactful moment of his life. Jason's father died in a car accident when Jason was six years old, and the death negatively affected the entire family. Jason's mother began to abuse prescription medications and would disregard Jason, leaving him in the house by himself for days on end. As he grew up, Jason developed his own substance-abuse habits and eventually began to use heroin. When discussing these events in treatment, Jason focused heavily on being abandoned by his parents; he saw himself as a victim of these events.

Because of his childhood, Jason developed a belief that anyone he grew close to would eventually leave him, and he had difficultly trusting others. Through his work in treatment, Jason also realized that he never fully grieved his father's death because his family members were very self-focused during that time. Jason, as a six-year-old, was still confused by death and did not have his family's support to help him grieve healthfully.

Jason began to recognize that, although he had been subject to very unfortunate circumstances in his childhood, he did not have to continue allowing them to rule his life. Jason recognized that the bitterness he had been holding onto was fueling his addiction and making it difficult to fully embrace sobriety. He began to look at other events in his life, too, and see how the way he viewed them created walls between him and a better life.

With help from his counselor, Jason worked diligently to explore his own grieving process and reconstruct how he viewed tragic moments from his life. He developed a new narrative—one of him as a survivor and a hero rather than a victim and a villain. This new view of self and story helped Jason come to peace with his past and start a new life.

FOR REFLECTION

• How has the death of a friend or family member affected your life? What emotions did you feel?

_____

_____

_____

_____

_____

• Aside from death, what are other life issues or events that can lead to the grieving process? Recall a time you've been through such an experience.

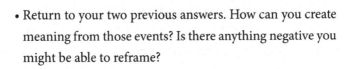

- Return to your two previous answers. How can you create meaning from those events? Is there anything negative you might be able to reframe?

CHAPTER ELEVEN

The Issue with Cross-Addiction

The term "cross-addiction" is the bogeyman of the recovery community: *Be careful doing that activity, because you might become addicted to it, too! Oh, no!* We are not trying to trivialize it, but the reverence with which people acknowledge cross-addiction can be a little intense. The belief behind cross-addiction is that once you are addicted to one substance, you are predisposed to becoming addicted to another substance or stimulating activity. Basically, because you're an addict to one, you're an addict to all, right?

Nope. We strongly believe that no one is "doomed" to a life of being perpetually addicted to all things because he or she has been addicted to one thing. We like to think that people can develop effective coping skills that will prevent further addictions. We also believe people can enjoy stimulating activities without fearing cross-addiction. And our beliefs come from reputable research. In this chapter, we will briefly review that research so you can be better informed.

At the same time, cross-addiction is not entirely impossible. It's been such a concern for so long for a reason. We'll also review some activities and non-narcotic substances that can be addictive. Let's get started.

So Cross-Addiction Isn't Real?

Not really. Until recently, the majority of information on cross-addiction did not come from research, but from case studies of individuals who either experienced this themselves or observed it happening to someone else. It made a lot of sense to see this happening and draw the conclusion of cross-addiction.

But let's look at the research, focusing on a study that came out in 2014 in *JAMA Psychiatry*. Researchers at Columbia University Medical Center surveyed 34,000 adults with substance-abuse disorders over the course of several years to determine whether they developed a new addiction. What they found was that people who were able to successfully cease use of their first substance were actually *less* likely to develop an addiction to another substance. People who *did* become addicted to another substance were ones who continued use of their original substance and did not successfully cease that use. In short, people who are able to successfully address the issues relevant to their substance use and remain sober are less likely to develop a cross-addiction.

When you break it down, this makes sense. If a person is able to remain sober, he or she has done a lot of beneficial work, such as addressing the problematic thoughts and behaviors associated with his or her addiction; developing healthy, effective coping skills; and establishing a sober support network. When someone has those things in place, he or she is less likely to develop another addiction because there is no longer a need or desire to rely on a substance. These individuals are not necessarily perfectly "cured," but they have the tools in place to live healthy and sober lives.

CROSS-ADDICTION AND BEHAVIORS

While the research mostly applies to cross-addiction with other substances, professionals in the field suggest that this also applies to addictive activities, such as gambling. If you've addressed your addictive behaviors with substances, you've addressed your addictive behaviors across the board. More research is needed on this specific area, though, and that is why we still want to talk about these activities. This is especially important in early recovery.

The research found that cross-addiction was less likely to occur with people who successfully addressed their addiction issues. Those in early recovery might fall into an addictive behavior that "replaces" their use before they're able to successfully resolve those problems and develop new coping skills. This is a common trap for many people in early recovery because they justify their behaviors by stating, "Well, at least I'm not using drugs!" The fact is that there are some activities that can be highly stimulating and also highly destructive if not kept in check.

Let's quickly clarify something. What do we mean when we say "stimulating"? With substance use, the reward centers of the brain are affected. When a substance is introduced to the brain, chemicals associated with pleasure and positive emotions rise to high levels, thus creating that "high" feeling. This is one factor that makes something addicting—the person's brain enjoys that elevated level and wants to experience it again.

Substances are not the only thing that elevates those levels, though. Plenty of daily activities cause those levels to rise and fall naturally. For instance, receiving a hug from a loved one raises those levels. So does watching a funny show or eating a delicious meal.

Some activities, though, are more stimulating than others and can be addicting in themselves. Therefore, people who have substance-use issues and have not fully addressed them might come to rely on these activities as a replacement. We are going to go over some of the main culprits and discuss why they should be on your radar. If you find yourself excessively engaging in any of these activities, it might be something to look at.

ALCOHOL

A common argument we hear among clients is whether a person whose substance of choice was a drug can drink alcohol without developing an issue. Clients will get into massive debates about this topic. And clients who are in treatment for alcohol-use disorder become flustered at the idea of someone who is addicted to drugs seeing alcohol as a "lesser evil."

But given the findings on cross-addiction, the research totally supports a cocaine addict's ability to drink, right? Maybe—and maybe not. We are not going to tell you that drinking is totally okay as long as you've addressed your issues related to addiction, and we are not going to tell you that you can never drink again. We believe in people making their own choices. We would encourage you to explore *why* you want to drink. What would drinking an alcoholic beverage do for you? What is the motivation behind taking the drink?

Some clients go on to eventually be able to have the occasional drink without it becoming a problem for them. Others find that drinking sparks a desire to use their original drug of choice. Many choose not to take the chance and instead abstain from all substances. It's all about personal choice and awareness of risks. Also, the research states that successful remission from the substance lessens the chance of cross-addiction. This does not apply to those new in recovery, and relying on alcohol instead of relying on drugs is not any healthier for you.

FOOD

Yep, something we need to survive also can be addictive. This is especially true for sugary foods; more and more research is being released that cites sugar as an addictive substance with tolerance and withdrawal symptoms. Eating itself is an activity that naturally stimulates the brain's pleasure centers, and it can provide a sense of comfort. Just think about it: Have you ever had a time when you felt emotional and then ate a lot of food? If you answered no, then teach us your secrets! Emotional eating is a common problem for many people, not just those who abuse substances. If you find yourself consistently turning to food in order to relieve stress, reward yourself, or provide a sense of happiness, that might be something to look at. Emotional eating can lead to excessive food consumption, which can be damaging to your health.

SEX AND PORNOGRAPHY

It goes without saying that sex is a highly stimulating activity—it has a major impact on the brain's pleasure center! Sex is not a bad thing, but like food, it can create problems for people if used in unhealthy ways. People in early recovery often struggle with developing healthy sex lives, because many of them initially explored their sexuality while under the influence. Now, as sober individuals, they are unsure how to pursue healthy sexual relationships with others. The emotions involved with sex also can be confusing, because re-exploration of emotions is a common pursuit in sobriety. Some people even begin to rely on sex as a coping mechanism or utilize it as a way to continue engaging in addictive behaviors.

The activities that lead up to sex—the desire, the search for a willing partner, the actual ritual leading up to and having sex, the quick release of positive emotion—are thought processes and behaviors similar to alcohol- and drug-seeking and use. The emotions following the action also can be similar: a sense of confusion and/or shame or a desire to re-engage in that "search" for satisfaction.

Many people also turn to pornography to satisfy that "craving" because it's easy to utilize and quickly satisfies that pleasure center. Pornography and sex addiction can cause major issues for people and their personal relationships. Pornography can create unrealistic views of sex and sexuality, and some people prefer to engage with pornography rather than with people due to its ease of "use."

If this is something you can relate to, we want to make it clear that there is nothing shameful about this. It's actually very common, and some clients might need to engage in post-treatment specific to sex and relationship issues in order to develop a healthier view of these things.

VIDEO GAMES AND TECHNOLOGY

Have you ever heard of people staying up for days on end, surviving on energy drinks, to play a video game? Maybe you've even done that yourself. We know this is an extreme example, but it does show how video games can be highly stimulating. It would be difficult to engage in an activity like that if it did not provide *something* pleasurable to the brain. Video games provide an escape from reality that is fun and engaging, and this can become an issue if not regulated. This can be especially true for games that have a social element. People might feel emotionally attached to the people they play with online, which can cause a detachment from real-life relationships. People can become preoccupied with their gaming and ignore their real-life responsibilities in order to participate. Does any of this sound familiar?

Another issue related to technology is social media and the Internet. We discussed social media and comparisons in chapter seven, so we've already established how dangerous social media can be. Social media also can be addicting, and many people struggle to distinguish their social media lives from their real lives. As with video games, people can become increasingly involved on social media and might ignore their real-life responsibilities and relationships in order to engage with the Internet. Microblogging is becoming more frequent, and some people feel a need to document and post many aspects of their lives online. Some people also develop meaningful relationships with others online. While this is not inherently bad, when taken to extremes it can cause problems in real life.

MONEY: SHOPPING AND GAMBLING

Many people new to sobriety express struggles with money management. After years of active addiction when the majority of their money went to their substance, having and saving money can be difficult. People in early recovery express issues with impulsive spending. This is probably caused by the association that having money equaled immediately spending it to get their fix. Now that substances are out of the picture, they still might feel a need to spend immediately and obtain a "fix" in the form of a new item or service. This causes many people to end up living paycheck to paycheck and being unable to afford their necessities. Proper budgeting and money management is a necessary skill for all people to learn, and it is especially important for those new to sobriety.

Gambling is also an activity to keep an eye on due to its addictive nature. Gambling can be an exciting activity. The thrill of the unknown, the rush whenever you get a win, the chances of leaving with more money than you entered with—it definitely activates that pleasure center. It also can be a destructive activity. People who become addicted to gambling often find themselves in terrible financial situations, struggling with interpersonal relationships, or facing legal trouble from stealing in order to have money to gamble. Preoccupation with gambling can cause a person to ignore his or her responsibilities and relationships. Are you seeing the pattern yet?

Gambling is slightly different from typical addictions, though, because it is more of a compulsion than a dependence. People who are addicted to gambling feel *compelled* to engage in that activity and feel anxious and uneasy until they are able to do so. It provides a thrill and an escape from reality. If you are new to sobriety, it might be smart to avoid the casino, Internet card games, and poker nights altogether, but if you are going to engage in gambling activities, make sure you set a limit and stick to it. If you don't think you can do that, then take a second to think about why you want to gamble in the first place.

Bringing It All Together

Though this chapter did not provide a comprehensive list of possibly addictive activities, we hope it provided some food for thought on how certain activities can affect the brain and its reward center. Drugs and alcohol are not the only things out there that can be problematic for people, and we hope that having an awareness can help you keep an eye on yourself and those around you. If you find yourself having issues with any of the things we discussed, there is help for *all* of those problems! Seek out a counselor or support system to assist you in learning how to engage in those activities in a healthy and productive way rather than in an excessive and destructive manner.

One thing we want to make very clear is that we are in no way saying people should not go shopping, have sex, or eat certain foods! Sometimes when we have these discussions with clients, they begin to engage in black-and-white thinking and decide to swear off these things. No way! That is not necessary. It's all about learning how to maintain balance and not spend too much time preoccupied or reliant upon one thing or activity. That might mean a lot of trial and error, and you might have days when you eat too much or spend way too much time playing a video game. There is no need to freak out and think you've fallen victim to cross-addiction. That's called being human. Learn from it, brush it off, and keep on moving.

• • • MARIE'S STORY • • •

While in treatment, Marie was a positive and helpful person. She made significant changes and addressed issues related to her addiction. She graduated successfully from the program and went into sober living.

Several weeks after her graduation, Marie met a man at a support meeting. They dated for several months, and Marie was smitten. But out of the blue, Marie's boyfriend broke up with her and began to date another girl who frequently attended the meetings. Marie was lost. Most of her post-treatment life had been spent with this man, and now Marie was unsure of what to do with her time. Marie also felt abandoned and unwanted, which diminished her self-esteem.

Marie began to chat with other men in the group, and she had sex with several of them. She found herself depressed when she wasn't talking or being with a man. She would go to meetings specifically to find someone to hook up with, but it never felt "right" afterward. She initially felt comfort and relief, but then she felt ashamed. Marie began to view herself in a negative light and found herself anxious when alone.

Marie eventually began using again and returned to treatment after several hellish months. While back in treatment, Marie processed how her relationship had replaced the coping skills she had developed in treatment, and when that relationship no longer existed, she continued to rely on men. Marie worked to process her shame and developed a more positive sense of self. She recognized that sex was not the issue—it was her reliance on attention from men.

Marie graduated again, feeling more assured and determined not to enter into a relationship until she felt stable within herself. She is doing well today.

FOR REFLECTION

- How does knowing about current research affect your thinking about cross-addiction?

  _____

  _____

  _____

  _____

- Think of some things you enjoy doing. How can you ensure that you set limits for yourself and keep an appropriate balance in your life?

  _____

  _____

  _____

  _____

- What are some underlying issues of substance abuse that might translate to someone becoming addicted to food, sex, or gambling?

  _____

  _____

  _____

  _____

CHAPTER TWELVE

Frequently Asked Questions

Can't I or my loved one just stop using? What's the big deal?
Unfortunately that's not how it works. By the time an addiction becomes an addiction, there is a reliance upon the substance. To put it simply, the person's brain has been "rewired" by the substance, and work needs to be done to set it straight. Obviously, this is much more complicated than this brief answer, and we encourage you to read through this book (especially chapter one) to get a better grasp on addiction and its components. In the meantime, though, start eradicating that belief that the solution is telling someone, "Just stop it!" Although there are some people out there who have been able to "just stop it," that is not the reality for everyone.

Okay, so I need help. What type of treatment do I need? Do I really need to go to "rehab"?
Yay! Recognizing the need for help is a wonderful first step! The type of treatment you need is dependent upon a lot of factors, though. We recommend that you take a look at chapter two, in which we detail some options and offer some

insights on each one. The best way to determine which type of treatment might be appropriate for you, though, is to seek out a clinician or a social services agency and have an assessment done. They then can recommend options to you and connect you to resources. And yes, you might need to go to "rehab" (we prefer "residential treatment"), and that's okay. A huge mistake many people make is not pursuing the best treatment option(s) for them because it's a big change and it's scary. Don't hold yourself back. Take the leap!

Why do I have to follow some type of program? Isn't my addiction unique to me?

Sort of. The reasons you use, specific issues that contributed to or resulted from your use, and the way you process things are unique to you, yes. But addiction itself is pretty cut and dried: a reliance upon a substance or substances. As you can see in our chapter about treatment types, there are various ways to approach treating addiction, but again, even those are pretty similar: promote abstinence from substances, address issues related to use, and then make positive changes to support sobriety. If you find yourself thinking your addiction is so different and unique that there isn't a treatment option out there for you, then honestly, you might be using that as an excuse to continue using.

Will my brain ever go back to "normal"?

Yes and no. Here's the obvious part: Drugs and alcohol have a major impact on the brain and its functions. The unknown parts are exactly how and to what extent drugs and alcohol have affected *your* brain. That depends in part on the types or combinations of substances you used. Research provides a promising outlook, though, and overall it suggests that those who maintain long-term abstinence from substances see improvement (and usually a complete return) of their brain functions.

Will the cravings and urges ever go away?

Maybe. Again, it all depends on the person. Cravings and urges are a totally normal thing, and it's also totally normal to have them on occasion even after weeks, months, or years of sobriety. As we said, the brain is changed by addiction. After years of dependence on a substance, the brain isn't going to let go that easily. It will take time for cravings to go away, but they will eventually. As you take steps away from using and learn new coping skills, the urges and cravings will lessen. When they do occur, try to see it as an opportunity to learn how to cope with them in a healthy way. Rather than see it as a weakness or a sign that you aren't "getting better," see it as your brain healing and as part of pursuing a better life.

I keep hearing about "ninety meetings in ninety days." Do I have to do that?

A lot of clients ask us this question, and we usually don't give a direct reply because we want people to explore their own options. We bring in several types of support groups at our treatment centers so people can explore which ones, if any, might be helpful for them post-treatment. If you want to pursue a ninety-in-ninety because you believe it will be beneficial to your sobriety, then great! Try it out! Here's the thing, though: You also need to be realistic. Do you have the ability to accomplish this goal? If life happens one day and prevents you from making it to a meeting, will that cause you major distress? The issue that sometimes occurs with ninety-in-ninety is that all-or-nothing thinking creeps in. People will miss a meeting and feel ashamed or like they failed rather than recognizing the reality of the situation: Life happens, mistakes happen, and ninety-in-ninety is a choice, not a requirement, for sobriety.

Do I have to go to sober living?
That's for you to decide. Entering into sober living can be a highly beneficial decision, but that does not mean it's necessary for everyone. Many people choose to go to sober living in order to place themselves in an environment with structure and accountability. It might be a good choice if your previous environment is not a healthy one, or if you're looking to surround yourself with people in the same boat. Not all sober-living facilities are the same, though. Definitely check them out and research their policies before you make a choice.

Is it okay to be in a relationship early in recovery?
This is a two-part answer. The first part is for those who are already in a relationship. If you are in a relationship while

in active addiction, a lot of work probably will need to be done when entering into sobriety. Whether both of you were in addiction or not, addiction brings toxicity into relationships that will need to be addressed. This might mean improving communication, ceasing enabling (see chapter one), addressing a lack of trust, and so on. Really look at the relationship and your feelings toward it. Also, don't fall into the trap of staying together just to stay together. If it's not working, forcing it will just make things more toxic.

For those of you who are single and looking to mingle, here's our take on it: We are not going to throw out a timeline of when you can be in a relationship. What we can say, though, is that you might want to ask yourself some questions. What are your intentions for entering into a relationship? Are you currently supporting yourself both emotionally and financially? Are you able to deal with conflict in healthy ways? Do you have goals? Will entering into a relationship jeopardize any of those goals? What we tend to see in early recovery is that people enter into relationships quickly because it allows them to focus on someone besides themselves. It also satisfies the codependency that often comes with addiction. So be honest with yourself. And if you can't do that, maybe a relationship isn't the best choice right now.

Can I still hang around my old friends?

We get this question a lot, and it baffles us. We know it's difficult to accept, but hanging around old friends with whom you used to use is probably one of the worst decisions you can make. Hanging out with people who are still in active addiction will only keep you in that lifestyle. Even if you don't directly use, you're surrounding yourself with what you are trying to get away from. Take a peek at chapter seven to see some more thoughts on this, especially in regards to connections on social media.

Okay, so what if they got sober as well? That might be okay, but we've seen many people have issues with this, especially if the thought patterns and behaviors associated with using are still present. Many times people forget about the reality of the past and focus on "the good ol' days" when hanging out with old using friends, and it can lead to some dangerous thoughts and/or actions. Be selective about the people with whom you surround yourself. Don't hang out with old "friends" just because it's comfortable and easy. Unfortunately, pursuing a sober life is not always comfortable and easy, but it is worth it. The relationships you form in sobriety will be much more meaningful and supportive than any based on substance use.

My loved one is in early recovery. How can I best support him?

First things first—listen to the person. *Really* listen to him, without any preconceived notions or beliefs. Let your loved one communicate with you about his thoughts and feelings without judgment. Utilize empathy and understanding to bridge connections. This might be hard, because you might not entirely understand where he is coming from. You might even have difficulty grasping the concept of addiction, and that's okay. Seeking to better understand is a great step in supporting someone. Maybe even ask how you can support your loved one, how you can help when he is struggling. The truth is, your loved one will struggle, and having a solid and nonjudgmental support system is a wonderful asset in sobriety.

Now, we want to make it clear that we don't associate "support" with "money." We are talking about emotional support here. Your monetary support is entirely up to you, and we encourage you to set boundaries with it.

That leads us to this advice: Take care of yourself! Addiction is not a single-person issue; it extends outward. Your loved one living with addiction probably had a huge effect on you. Looking at your own issues and the stresses that arose during that time will be very helpful for you. Seeking out counseling and support groups for families and significant others of addicts could be a great step, in addition to possibly seeking out individual counseling. Addressing your own issues so you and your loved one can grow together is another great way to be supportive.

Websites

SAMHSA.gov—The Substance Abuse and Mental Health Services Administration has educational materials on addiction and mental health.

CDC.gov—The Centers for Disease Control and Prevention website offers statistics and other helpful medical information about alcohol and drug abuse.

DrugAbuse.gov—The National Institute on Drug Abuse provides research-based facts and information about addiction.

NAMI.org—The National Alliance on Mental Illness website includes information and resources for seeking help and support.

AA.org—The Alcoholics Anonymous website provides information about AA and how to find meetings in your area.

NA.org—The Narcotics Anonymous website provides information about NA and how to find meetings in your area.

Al-anon.alateen.org—Al-Anon provides support for family members and loved ones of problem drinkers.

Nar-anon.org—Nar-Anon provides support for family members and loved ones of those struggling with addiction.

SmartRecovery.org—The website provides information about SMART Recovery and how to find meetings in your area.

CelebrateRecovery.com—The website provides information about Celebrate Recovery, which is a Christ-centered program, and how to find meetings in your area.

Books and articles

American Psychiatric Association. *Diagnostic and Statistical Manual of Mental Disorders (5th Edition)*. Washington, D.C.: American Psychiatric Publishing, 2013.

Blanco, C., Okuda, M., Wang, S., Liu, S., and Olfson, M. (2014). "Testing the Drug Substitution Switching-Addictions Hypothesis." *JAMA Psychiatry*, 71(11), 1246. doi:10.1001/jamapsychiatry.2014.1206

Foote, Jeffrey, Carrie Wilkens, Nicole Kosanke, and Stephanie Higgs. *Beyond Addiction: How Science and Kindness Help People Change*. New York: Scribner, 2014.

Frankl, Viktor. *Man's Search for Meaning*. Boston: Beacon Press, 2006.

Glasner-Edwards, Suzette. *The Addiction Recovery Skills Workbook: Changing Addictive Behaviors Using CBT, Mindfulness, and Motivational Interviewing Techniques*. Oakland, Calif.: New Harbinger Publications, 2016.

James, John W. and Russell, Friedman. *The Grief Recovery Handbook: 20th Anniversary Edition*. N.p.: HarperCollins, 2009.

Kübler-Ross, Elisabeth. *On Death and Dying: What the Dying Have to Teach Doctors, Nurses, Clergy and Their Own Families*. London: Routledge, 2009.

Sheff, David. *Beautiful Boy: A Father's Journey Through His Son's Addiction*. New York: Mariner, 2008.

Spiegelman, Erica. *Rewired: A Bold New Approach to Addiction and Recovery*. Hobart, New York: Hatherleigh Press, 2015.

Williams, Rebecca E., and Julie S. Kraft. *The Mindfulness Workbook for Addiction: A Guide to Coping with the Grief, Stress, and Anger that Trigger Addictive Behaviors*. Oakland, Calif.: New Harbinger Publications, 2012.

Additional books by KiCam Projects

Adams Recovery Center. *Addiction, Recovery, Change: A How-To Manual for Successfully Navigating Sobriety*. Georgetown, Ohio: KiCam Projects, 2016.

Leder, Sharon. *The Fix: A Father's Secrets, A Daughter's Search*. Georgetown, Ohio: KiCam Projects, 2017.

Also available from KiCam Projects:

Addiction, Recovery, Change
*A How-To Manual for Successfully
Navigating Sobriety*
by ADAMS RECOVERY CENTER

Whether you're building a new life
or supporting a loved one, this is
the resource you need to meet the
everyday challenges of staying clean
and sober.

$11.95 / 112 pages

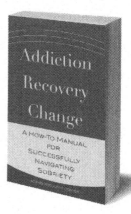

The Fix
*A Father's Secrets,
A Daughter's Search*
by SHARON LEDER

Through the eyes of Sara Katz,
author Sharon Leder makes peace
with her family's history as she
explores her childhood as the
daughter of a heroin addict who lost
his battle with drugs.

$19.95 / 256 pages

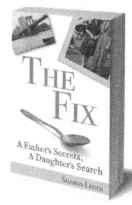

Available now on KiCamProjects.com and Amazon.com.

To learn more about Adams Recovery Center,
please visit AdamsRecoveryCenter.org,
call 513-575-0968,
or email info@adams-recovery-center.org.